Clinical Handbook

HEALTH ASSESSMENT IN NURSING

Sims · D'Amico
Stiesmeyer · Webster

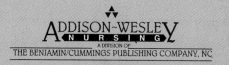

ADDISON-WESLEY
NURSING
A DIVISION OF
THE BENJAMIN/CUMMINGS PUBLISHING COMPANY, INC.

Redwood City, California · Menlo Park, California
Reading, Massachusett · New York · Don Mills, Ontario
Wokingham, U.K. · Amsterdam · Bonn · Sydney
Singapore · Tokyo · Madrid · San Juan

Executive Editor: Patricia L. Cleary
Acquisitions Editor: Erin Mulligan
Editorial Consultant: Tom Lochhaas
Project Editor: Grace Wong
Production Supervisor: Larry Olsen
Designer and Compositor: Richard Kharibian
Art Coordinator: Janice Gaal
Cover Designer: Yvo Riezebos
Cover photo: Carina Woolrich, San Diego, California
Cover quilt: Spring: Garden Series #1, by Glenne Stoll

Care has been taken to confirm the accuracy of information presented in this book. The
authors, editors, and the publisher, however, cannot accept any responsibility for errors or
omissions or for the consequences from application of the information in this book and make
no warranty, express or implied, with respect to its contents.

The authors and publisher have exerted every effort to ensure that drug selections and
dosages set forth in this text are in accord with current recommendation and practice at time
of publication. However, in view of ongoing research, changes in government regulations,
and the constant flow of information relating to drug therapy and drug reactions, the reader
is urged to check the package inserts of all drugs for any change in indications of dosage and
for added warnings and precautions. This is particularly important when the recommended
agent is a new and/or infrequently employed drug.

ISBN 0-8053-7349-7

1 2 3 4 5 6 7 8 9 10—BA—99 98 97 96 95

Library of Congress Cataloging-in-Publication Data

Clinical handbook to accompany health assessment in nursing / Sims ... (et al.).
    p.   cm.
    Includes index.
    ISBN 0-8053-7349-7
    1. Nursing assessment—Handbooks, manuals, etc.   2. Physical
    diagnosis—Handbooks, manuals, etc.   I. Sims, Lina K.   I. Health
    assessment in nursing.
    (DNLM: 1. Nursing assessment—handbooks.   2. Medical History
    Taking—nurses' instruction—handbooks.   3. Physical Examination—
    nurses' instruction—handbooks.   4. Interview, Psychological—nurses'
    instruction—handbooks.   WY 49 1995)
    RT48.H446   1995 Suppl.
    616.07′5—dc20
    DNLM/DLC   94-45761
                                                                              CIP

Addison-Wesley Nursing
A Division of The Benjamin/Cummings Publishing Company, Inc.
390 Bridge Parkway
Redwood City, California 94065

Contents

Preface

The *Clinical Handbook* is a pocket-sized reference guide designed to help both nursing students and practicing nurses in their assessment of clients. It contains information on the complete health assessment, including both the focused health history and the key elements of the physical examination.

Chapters 1 to 4 introduce the principles and techniques that are the foundation of the holistic health assessment. You will learn to conduct an effective interview and health history, organize gathered data, focus on psychosocial health, and assess vital signs. These chapters also review the basic examination skills, general survey procedures, and universal precautions.

Chapters 5 to 15 present the physical assessment by body system. Each chapter contains the following features:

- A list of specific "Focused Interview" questions
- A "Physical Assessment" section, which includes step-by-step descriptions of how to perform the physical examination, presented in a two-column format to distinguish between normal findings and special considerations
- "Alerts" and "Referrals" in red where special circumstances call for modification of the assessment procedure or immediate medical attention
- Photographs and line art to illustrate key assessment steps and findings
- Lists of "Nursing Diagnoses" and "Common Alterations" related to each body system
- A "Client Education" section that provides specific suggestions for health promotion and disease prevention
- A "Physical Assessment Summary," which provides a quick review of body system assessment

Chapters 16 to 18 provide a head-to-toe assessment for three special client populations: infants, children, and adolescents, the childbearing client, and the older adult.

The *Clinical Handbook* is ideal as a companion guide for nursing students who are using a full-length health assessment text such as *Health Assessment in Nursing* by Sims, D'Amico, Stiesmeyer, and Webster, or as a reference guide for practicing nurses who have completed their basic training.

Chapter 1

Health Assessment: Interview and Health History

Health assessment is a systematic method of collecting data about a client to determine his or her health status. During the health assessment interview, the client will tell you about events and experiences related to his or her current state of health. You will also explore clients' concerns, emotions, expectations, and knowledge about their health. Information gained from the assessment can be used to help the client prevent illness, maintain health, and cure disease.

Using a Holistic Approach

In health assessment, using a holistic approach means considering all aspects of a client's health in relation to the health problem in order to help the client move toward optimal health. In addition to assessing a client's physiologic health status in relation to the current health problem, you take into consideration:

- **Additional health factors**—factors that may seem unrelated to the client's present problem, but that can yield information affecting the progress or outcome of the assessment
- **Developmental factors**—client's developmental stage
- **Psychosocial factors**—client's emotional health, level of stress and anxiety, and general satisfaction with life
- **Self-care factors**—factors related to client's health practices, including nutrition, exercise, hygiene, and grooming; use of tobacco, alcohol, and other drugs; safety practices; and rest and recreation
- **Family, cultural and environmental factors**—client's family structure, cultural group, religious practices, socioeconomic status, educational level, job, and living environment

Establishing the Nurse–Client Relationship

Clients are more willing to discuss their health issues with you if they feel that that there is mutual trust and understanding. Some characteristics that establish trust include:

- **Positive regard**—appreciate and respect the client's individuality, race, culture, and religion, with a nonjudgmental attitude
- **Empathy**—understand and support the client's feelings and experiences through actions and words
- **Genuineness**—present yourself honestly and spontaneously by focusing on the situation at hand
- **Concreteness**—speak to the client in specific terms rather than in vague generalities

Communication Skills for Health Assessment

Communication skills play an important role in developing a nurse-client relationship, in conducting the health assessment interview, and in collecting data for the health history. Following are some hints for what to try and what to avoid when communicating with a client.

Aids to Nurse–Client Communication

- **Listening**—an active process that requires hearing the client's words as well as interpreting body language. Attentive listening involves encouraging the client to speak and paraphrasing a client's words to make sure you have understood the client accurately.
- **Leading**—includes direct leading, focusing, and questioning the client in order to start an interaction or to get the client to discuss specific health concerns
- **Reflecting**—occurs when you show a client that you empathize or are in tune with the client's thoughts, feelings, and experiences
- **Summarizing**—the process of gathering ideas, feelings, and themes that clients have discussed throughout the interview and restating them in several general statements. Summarizing shows clients that you have listened and understood their concerns and that progress is being made in resolving their concerns.

Barriers to Nurse–Client Communication

- **False reassurance**—assuring the client of a positive outcome with no basis for believing in it, which robs the client of the right to communicate his or her feelings

- **Interrupting or changing the subject**—shows insensitivity to the client's thoughts and feelings
- **Passing judgment**—making judgmental statements conveys a strong message that the client must live up to your value system to be accepted and discourages further interaction
- **Cross-examining**—"grilling" the client with an endless barrage of questions may cause the client to feel threatened and reveal less and less information. Help clients feel more at ease by encouraging them to express their feelings about the pace and nature of the interview.
- **Using technical terms**—instead, use lay terms rather than technical jargon whenever possible

Cultural Considerations

Differences in culture, ethnicity, religion, nationality, and language can affect the way a message is encoded and decoded. Following are some tips for effective communication when these differences arise:

- Be careful not to bring cultural stereotypes to the communication process.
- Learn as much as possible about the culture, values, and beliefs of your clients by asking and observing them and their families.
- Be aware that if you and your client are from different cultures, your body language may become an even more critical part of the communication process.
- Attempt to individualize communications styles to ethnic groups, but do not make assumptions about the ethnicity of clients. Differences among individuals in a group are often greater than the differences between groups.
- If a client does not speak the same language, have a translator assist with the interview.
- If your client communicates better with the written word, have pencil and paper readily available.

Developing the Database

The first step in health assessment is developing the database, which involves collecting information about a client that may hint at possible health problems. The database is collected during the initial client interview, the focused interview, and the physical assessment. Database content includes information about the client's health patterns, self-care activities, activities of daily living, wellness concerns, past health history, current health issues, and other aspects of the client's health status.

The source of data is *primary* (client) or *secondary* (eg, family, friends, health personnel, medical records, literature). Data can be *objective* (observable or measurable) or *subjective* (symptoms), *constant* or *variable*. Accuracy of both objective and subjective data can be increased through use of clarifying questions, supporting data, verification, and attention to detail.

The focused interview is used to uncover additional information related to a specific health problem. Though it should always occur before a physical assessment, it can also be used at any point during the physical assessment to gain more information about signs or symptoms.

The physical assessment is the hands-on assessment of the client to confirm the absence of health problems or to uncover unexpected findings.

Guidelines for Conducting a Health Assessment Interview

1. Provide a setting that is quiet, private, free from distractions, and comfortable for the client.
2. Address the client by family name unless he or she gives you permission to use a given name.
3. Explain the purpose of the interview before beginning to ask questions. Use a calm, friendly, unhurried approach, and allow clients enough time to answer at their own pace.
4. Communicate at the client's level of understanding, considering their age, sex, level of education, and culture when formulating assessment questions.
5. Use open, attending body language that conveys your interest and concern.
6. Make brief notations as you question the client. Use a predetermined format to record data if available.
7. Interview a close family member, friend, or significant other if the client is unable to communicate.
8. Use terminology that the client understands. Avoid jargon, slang, and clichés.

Permission and Validation

Whenever possible, obtain the client's written or verbal permission before requesting information from another person. Also, be cautious when collecting client data from other people, since it may be prejudiced by their personal biases, life experiences, and values. Try to validate it with at least one other source, especially when it conflicts with information provided by the client.

Phases of the Health Assessment Interview

The health assessment interview is divided into three phases: preinteraction, initial interview, and focused interview. The first two phases provide information you use along with the physical assessment to develop the client database, formulate nursing diagnoses, and initiate the nursing care plan. The focused interview occurs throughout all stages of the nursing process and is a tool to help you gather, clarify, and update additional client data as it becomes available. Table 1.1 provides a breakdown of the phases and associated activities.

TABLE 1.1   Phases of the Health Assessment Interview

Phase	Activities
Phase I **Preinteraction**	Gather data from medical records, other health personnel. Review relevant literature. Plan the setting and time for the initial interview.
Phase II **Initial interview**	Establish a nurse-client relationship. Describe the purposes of the interview. Interview the client. Document health history data. Validate data with secondary sources if necessary. Use information to plan the physical exam.
Phase III **Focused interview**	Collect data supporting hypothesized nursing, medical, or collaborative diagnoses. Clarify previously obtained data. Gather data that is new or missing. Update information about specific health problems.

The Health History

The nursing health history is a complete record of the client's past and current health status. It is gathered during the initial health assessment interview, usually at the client's first visit to a health care facility. The purpose of the nursing health history is to document the response of the whole person to actual and potential health concerns.

The goal of the interview process is to obtain information about the client's health status. The information from the nursing health history, along with the subsequent data from the physical assessment, is used to develop a set of nursing diagnoses that reflect the client's health concerns.

Organization of the Health History

Most health care settings have health history forms for collecting data, organizing it, and ensuring that the interviewer does not omit any information. The organization of the health history form differs among health care settings. However, all health history models focus on the current health concern, along with an additional broad focus on all aspects of the client's lifestyle and response to the environment. In general, health histories include the following groups of information:

Biographic Data

Full name (including maiden name if female, mother's maiden name if male), age and birth date, place of birth, sex, race, nationality, culture and ethnicity, marital status, family members and significant others living with client, contact person's name and address, occupation, address, telephone number, Social Security number, religion, education level, insurance coverage.

Reason for Seeking Care and History of Present Health Concern

Why are you seeking care? How do you feel about having to seek care? What medications or treatments have you used? How effective were they? What aggravates this health concern? What alleviates symptoms? What caused the health concern to occur? How has the concern affected life and daily activities? Onset of the concern, duration of the concern, course of the health concern, signs, symptoms, and related behavior, previous history and episodes of this condition, related health concerns, expectations for recovery, expectations for self-care.

Client Health History

Birth history, growth and development history, immunization history, childhood diseases, allergies, previous health concerns, previous hospitalizations, surgical procedures, pregnancies and deliveries, accidents and injuries, blood transfusions; emotional or psychiatric problems, ongoing medications, prescription medications, over-the-counter medications, recreational drugs, birth control use, vitamins, caffeine use, past alcohol use.

Be sure to record dates and, when pertinent, locations, treatment, health care providers, and type of surgery and postoperative care.

Family History (Genogram)

Age and health status of living grandparents, parents, siblings, children, aunts, uncles, and cousins; age and cause of death of deceased grandparents, parents, siblings, children, aunts, uncles, and cousins; any family history of heart disease, diabetes, obesity, lung disease, tuberculosis, mental illness, cancer, arthritis, genetic disorders, hypertension, or neurologic disease.

Review of Body Systems

Integumentary system, cardiovascular system, axillae and breasts, gastrointestinal system, urinary system, reproductive system, peripheral vascular system, musculoskeletal system, neurologic system, endocrine system.

Health Patterns

Nutrition, weight control, activity/fitness/exercise, sleep/rest, self-perception/body image/self-concept/self-esteem, role performance/relationship patterns, sexuality-reproduction/sexual responsibility/breast and testicular self-examination, coping, stress tolerance, locus of control, safety/accident prevention (home, work, driving), environmental hazards/exposure to air pollution, toxic chemicals, radiation, psychosocial/communication style, leisure and recreational activities, substance use, medical self-care.

Documenting the Data

The main purpose of documentation is accurate and thorough communication of the health assessment data to others involved in the client's care. All documentation should be clear, accurate, objective, specific, concise, and current. Clear, objective documentation also protects you, the client, and the health care agency, serving as legal proof and a permanent record of the client's health at the time.

What you choose to document depends on your client care objectives and information needs for formulating nursing diagnoses or planning nursing interventions. Learning how to identify physical cues and related factors for each body system will help you decide what to document and what to disregard.

When you have completed the health assessment and organized and documented the information obtained, communicate the data to the rest of the team members who provide care for the client.

Identifying Nursing Diagnoses

Nursing diagnoses are statements used by nurses to describe a client's response to health problems that nurses are educated about and licensed to treat. Identifying nursing diagnoses requires an ability to gather significant diagnostic data and draw logical conclusions from it. If you are still learning assessment and diagnostic skills, you may use the model outlined below until identifying nursing diagnoses becomes second nature.

1. Gather preliminary data.
   - Gather data from your initial interview of the client and significant others, medical records, and discussion with other health professionals. During the initial interview, take a health history.
   - If necessary, review the literature to research the expected norms for comparison with client data and relevant anatomy and physiology, to understand client data and explore probable nursing diagnoses.
   - Compile this information as part of a preliminary database, to be used as a baseline against which to compare future changes in the client's condition.

2. Formulate diagnostic hypotheses.
   - Compare client data to standards. If cue does not compare to an accepted standard, a diagnostic hypothesis may be developed. A cue that deviates from normal is a signal that the client is responding abnormally. Begin looking for other cues that commonly occur along with the cue you observed.
   - Make inferences. Use known or observed facts to draw conclusions about a condition that is not directly observable.
   - State the hypothesis in the form of a probable or possible nursing diagnosis.

3. Gather supporting data.
   Gather data to support or reject the diagnostic hypotheses by conducting a focused interview and performing a physical assessment.

4. Organize and cluster data.
   After gathering the supporting data, sort and group all diagnostic cues collected according to the defining characteristics of specific nursing diagnoses.

5. Select and validate nursing diagnoses.
   Determine the final nursing diagnoses by comparing each diagnostic cluster with the defining characteristics of your tentative nursing diagnosis. When the two sets of data match, you have validated the diagnosis.

6. Identify etiologic or related factors.

   Identify and include etiologic or related factors in the nursing diagnoses to confirm the validity of the chosen nursing diagnoses. (In most cases, you will already have collected and identified this information along with the diagnostic cues.)

Promoting Client Health and Wellness

Health assessment can be applied to health promotion and wellness as well as to disease prevention and treatment.

The Wellness Assessment

Carry out a wellness assessment by working with your client to examine positive adaptations and previously successful behaviors that contribute to optimal health and well-being. By using a wellness framework for health assessment, you can help the client take responsibility for his or her own health. Emphasize the client's personal strengths and ability to enhance health. Demonstrate that health promotion is a priority when assessing the client and providing care.

Possible Goals of a Wellness Assessment

1. Reinforcing and continuing health-promoting behaviors.
2. Preventing illness.
3. Identifying acute or chronic needs and problems.
4. Supporting the client in meeting death with dignity.
5. Promoting spiritual wellness.
6. Eliminating behavioral risk factors, such as the use of tobacco, alcohol, and other drugs, lack of exercise, and poor nutrition.

Possible Wellness Assessment Questions

1. What issues are you concerned with regarding your health?
2. How does your health concern affect you and your lifestyle?
3. What do you think you need to do to resolve this concern?
4. What health goals do you want to begin moving toward?
5. What do you see as your strengths?
6. How do you feel your care provider or nurse can help you?

Chapter 2

Assessing Psychosocial Health

Psychosocial functioning includes the way a person thinks, feels, acts, and relates to self and others; his or her ability to cope and tolerate stress; and his or her capacity for developing a value and belief system. When assessing psychosocial functioning, pay attention to how the client's psychosocial health affects physical health, and vice versa. Psychosocial factors can play a direct role in many physiologic disorders. Clients in a state of optimum psychological, social, and spiritual well-being have faster recovery rates, better response rates to treatment modalities, and in some cases, lower mortality rates. Types of psychosocial behaviors vary by developmental stage; this chapter focuses on the adult stage of development.

Factors Affecting Psychosocial Wellness

- **Self-concept**—the feelings and beliefs people hold about themselves at any given time
- **Roles and relationships**—the set of behaviors that society or significant others expect of an individual in a certain position
- **Stress and coping**—the individual's physical and emotional response to psychosocial or physical threats to safety, called stressors
- **Senses and cognition**—the ways an individual perceives and makes sense of the environment, and the logical sequencing of thoughts and feelings
- **Spiritual and belief systems**—an individual's relationship with a higher power or ideal that gives meaning to life

Gathering Data

Before the initial interview, gather information from medical records relating to past emotional or psychiatric problems as well as physiologic illnesses that may have affected the client's psychological or social functioning.

During the initial interview, gather more information about the client's social history. If you discover an area of heightened concern, you can focus on that area.

During the focused interview, use information obtained from the medical history, initial interview, and subsequent client interactions to help the client do a careful inventory of past and current psychosocial health status. You should also observe the client's general appearance, posture, gait, body language, facial expression, affect, and speech patterns.

When to Focus an Interview on Psychosocial Well-Being

You may want to focus on a client's psychosocial health if any of the following factors is evident:

- If a client's primary health concern is psychosocial in nature
- When the information you collect during the health history indicates psychosocial dysfunction
- If the client's behavior during the initial interview is anxious, depressed, erratic, or bizarre
- If you need more information to determine whether relationships exist between past disease processes and potential emotional or psychiatric concerns
- When an emotional problem becomes apparent later in a client's care—for example, when the client undergoes a disfiguring surgical procedure

Use the focused interview to collect information about the client's past history of psychosocial and physiological problems as well as the five areas of psychosocial functioning.

Past History of Psychosocial Concerns

Some psychosocial concerns begin early in life and reappear whenever a client faces a major stressor or life crisis. Information about the way a client coped with problems and treatment modalities in the past can be useful in planning for the client's current problems. The following questions may help to elicit such information:

1. Describe any emotions you find yourself frequently experiencing, both currently and in the past.

2. If you have had an emotional problem in the past, were you treated for it? What was the treatment, and was it successful? Who treated you and when? Do you still have the problem?

3. Do you use alcohol or drugs? Which ones, how much, and how often? Have you been treated for substance abuse? What was the treatment? Where were you treated?

4. Have you had any eating problems such as anorexia or bulimia? Were you treated? How? By whom? When?

Past and Current History of Physiologic Alterations or Diseases

Clients may be unaware that their physical problems may be related to or caused by an underlying psychosocial problem. Ask the following questions to uncover additional information:

1. Describe any chronic illnesses you have had.

2. How has your illness changed your mood or feelings? When you are nervous or anxious, how does your body feel?

3. Have you had arthritis, asthma, bowel disorders, glandular problems, heart problems, headaches, stomach ulcers, or skin disorders? If so, describe how the condition has affected your life.

Self-Concept

Because most people are uneasy talking about themselves, establish a positive nurse–client relationship before trying to gather this information. It is best to try to integrate your questions into a general conversation.

1. How would you describe yourself to others?

2. What are your best characteristics? What do you like about yourself?

3. What would you change about yourself if you could?

4. Do you consider yourself attractive? Sexually appealing? If no, why not?

5. Have your feelings about your appearance changed with this illness? If so, how?

6. Who comes first in your life: your spouse, children, friends, parents, or yourself?

7. Do you have difficulty saying no to others?

8. Do you like to be alone?

9. Describe your social life. What do you do for fun?

10. Are you comfortable with your sexual preference? If no, why not?

11. Do you have any concerns about your sexual function? If so, what?

Family History

Explore family history more fully if the health history indicates a family history of psychosocial dysfunction. Explore individual as well as family dysfunction. Ask the following questions in relation to a client's current family:

1. Describe any problems your family may have had with mental disorders.
2. Describe your relationships with your parents and extended family.
3. What is your birth order in your family? How many siblings?
4. Describe your relationship with your siblings growing up at home. Did you have problems getting along? If so, how did you solve them?
5. What members of your extended family (grandparents, aunts, uncles, cousins) were important to you as you grew up? How did they influence you?
6. Did you have death or losses in your family as you grew up? How did your parents teach you to cope with the loss? How did they cope with the loss?
7. Were your parents divorced and/or remarried during your childhood? If so, with whom did you live? Describe your life growing up with a single parent or step-parent.
8. Describe how your parents raised you. How did it affect you?
9. How did your family deal with adversity and conflict?
10. When disagreement arose in your family, how was it solved? Who sided with whom?

Other Roles and Relationships

1. Describe your relationships with your friends, neighbors, and co-workers.
2. Do you belong to any social groups? Community groups?
3. Who is your closest friend? How do you maintain your friendship?
4. Is your closest friend the most important person in your life? If not, who is the most important person in your life? Explain why.

Stress and Coping

Depending upon how an individual copes with stress, he or she may be more likely to experience stress-related disorders such as headaches, asthma, skin rashes, back pain, frequent colds, and anxiety. Ask the following questions when gathering information about a client's stress and coping mechanisms:

1. What do you do for relaxation? For recreation?

2. What is your greatest source of comfort when you are upset?

3. Whom do you call when you need help?

4. What is the greatest source of stress in your life at the present time? How have you coped with similar situations in the past?

5. Describe how you are dealing with your illness. Have you had difficulty adjusting to changes in your appearance, ability to carry out activities of daily living, or relationships? If so, describe how you feel.

6. Do you take any drugs or medications or drink alcohol to cope with your stress? If so, describe them.

7. Are you experiencing any of the following?

Sadness	Loss of sex drive	Indecisiveness
Crying spells	Constipation	Confusion
Insomnia	Fatigue	Pounding heart or pulse
Lack of appetite	Hopelessness	Trouble concentrating
Weight loss	Irritability	

8. Have you ever considered taking your life? If so, describe what you would do. (Clients are at a high risk for suicide if they can describe a method and have the means at their disposal.)

The Senses and Cognition

Clients who are out of contact with reality may display illusional, delusional, and hallucinatory speech and behavior. Direct questioning may increase the client's anxiety, escalate abnormal behavior, or cause confusion. Question directly only when the client appears to be in control and in touch with reality. Before asking the following questions, explain to the client that while some of the questions may seem silly or unimportant, they are helpful in assessing memory.

1. What is your name, age, and place of birth?

2. Where are you right now?

3. What day of the week is it? What is the date?

4. What would you do if a fire broke out? (This evaluates the client's ability to make a judgment.)

5. Count backwards from 10 to 1.

6. What did you have for breakfast?

7. Who were the last two presidents?

8. Describe what the following statement means: "People who live in glass houses shouldn't throw stones." (This tests the client's ability to perform abstract and/or symbolic thinking.)

9. Are you having any problems thinking? If so, describe what happens.

10. Do you have trouble making decisions? Describe what happens when you have to make a decision.

11. Do you ever hear voices, see objects, or experience other sensations that don't make sense? If so, describe your experiences.

Spiritual and Belief Systems

The questions in this section determine how clients' ethical, moral, and religious values affect their health status. Often the client's statements about values play an important role in how you should implement nursing care.

1. Describe your ethnic and cultural background.

2. To whom do you go for help regarding your health (doctor, nurse practitioner, folk healer, medicine man, other healer)?

3. What are your beliefs about life, health, illness, and death?

4. Does religion or God play a part in your life? If so, what is it?

5. Do your spiritual beliefs help you cope with illness or stress? If so, describe how.

6. Have you experienced any anger with God or a higher being or force because of things that have happened to you? If so, describe how you feel.

7. Do you believe your illness is a punishment for past sins or wrong-doing?

8. If you use prayer, describe how it helps you cope with life or stress.

9. Describe any religion-related nutrition or health practices that you must follow.

10. Are you concerned about the morality or ethical implications of any of the treatments planned for you?

Organizing the Data

Once you have collected the data from the various sources, sort, group, and categorize the information under one of the following psychosocial functioning groups:

Self-Concept Group

Place a diagnostic cue in this group if it gives information about how the client feels about self, how the client thinks other people feel about or see him or her, or how the client is able to control his or her life.

Possible nursing diagnoses include Anxiety, Body-image disturbance, Hopelessness, Powerlessness, and Low self-esteem.

Roles and Relationships Group

Place a diagnostic cue in this group if it gives information about family relationships and dynamics, the client's relationships with others, or the client's support systems.

Possible nursing diagnoses include Altered family processes, Dysfunctional grieving, Parental role conflict, and Social isolation.

Stress and Coping Group

Place a diagnostic cue in this group if it gives information about sources of stress in the client's life, coping strategies and reactions to stressors (signs and symptoms); the client's use of chemical substances; losses of family or friends through death; other losses, such as loss of job or money; or signs and symptoms of depression or suicidal ideation.

Possible nursing diagnoses include Impaired adjustment, Ineffective individual coping, Ineffective family coping, Rape-trauma syndrome, and Potential for violence.

Sensory and Cognition Group

Place a diagnostic cue in this group if it gives information about reality orientation, thinking processes, or affective behavior.

Possible nursing diagnoses include Decisional conflict, Sensory/perceptual alterations, and Altered thought processes.

Spiritual Belief Group

Place a diagnostic cue in this group if it gives information about a relationship with a higher power, religious life, or a belief system.

Possible nursing diagnosis is Spiritual distress.

Identifying Nursing Diagnoses

After you have grouped and clustered the diagnostic cues under one of the five psychosocial groups, determine final nursing diagnoses. Compare each cluster to the defining characteristics of each diagnosis in the group until you determine an appropriate fit.

Chapter 3

Assessing Self-Care and Environmental Factors

Factors Affecting Physical Wellness

Self-Care and Wellness Activities

A client's wellness is greatly influenced by his or her personal health behaviors. During an assessment, you will want to collect data about a client's lifestyle and health practices in five major areas: activities of daily living (ADLs), nutrition, sleep and rest, exercise, and safety. Having assessed these areas, you will be able to:

1. Help the client determine the impact of his or her present activities on health and wellness.
2. Educate the client about health behaviors and lifestyle changes and develop a plan that he or she can use to maintain or increase the current level of wellness. Remember, however, that it is the client's responsibility to implement the plan.

Activities of Daily Living

Gather data on ADLs to determine whether the client is able to use daily living skills independently. If the client needs assistance for some or all activities, determine whether assistance is available. If the client is unable to function independently, alternate living arrangements may be needed. You can assess ADLs most successfully by observing the client in the home. If you must conduct the assessment elsewhere, request a client history to supplement your observations. Ask the following questions to gather data on the client's ability to perform basic ADLs:

Bathing/hygiene skills

1. Describe how you bathe or wash yourself.
2. Describe any problems you have getting out of the shower or bath.

3. What safety equipment do you have available when taking a bath (bath stool, nonslip mat)?
4. Describe any assistance you need in bathing or washing.
5. Are you able to wash your hair?
6. After you have bathed, are you able to dry yourself completely?

Mobility and transfer skills

1. Are you able to get up from a sitting or lying position without assistance?
2. Are you able to move around in bed without assistance?
3. Are you able to sit down in a chair without assistance?
4. Are you able to walk without assistance? Do you have any discomfort when you walk? Short distances? Long distances?
5. Do you use a cane, walker, or other assistive device to walk? How far are you able to walk with assistance?
6. Are you able to climb stairs or steps without assistance? If you have difficulty climbing stairs, describe it.
7. Do you use a prosthesis? How long have you used it?
8. Do you use a wheelchair?

Dressing skills

1. Are you able to select your clothing and get it out of the closet or drawer without assistance?
2. Are you able to put on your clothing without difficulty?
3. Describe any difficulty you have with buttons, zippers, or other fasteners on clothing. Do you have difficulty tying your shoelaces or buckling your shoes?
4. If you require assistance in dressing or undressing, describe the amount and type of assistance needed.

Grooming skills

1. Do you have difficulty brushing, combing, or styling your hair? Do you need assistive devices (eg, built-up brush handles)?
2. If you wear makeup, do you have any difficulty applying it?
3. Are you able to shave? If not, who shaves you?
4. Are you able to wash, iron, fold, and maintain your clothes?

Eating skills

1. Are you able to prepare your own meals? If not, where do you eat or how do you get your food?
2. Describe any problems you may have feeding yourself.

3. Describe any difficulty you have in chewing or swallowing your food, including solids and liquids. Does food or drink get caught in your throat?

4. Do you require any assistance for eating? Do you use any assistive devices (eg, built-up handles)? Describe the type and amount of assistance needed.

Shopping skills

1. Are you able to get to and walk through the store to shop for food, clothing, and other basic needs?

2. Are you able to select the items that you need?

3. Are you able to carry your purchases home?

4. Do you require any assistance for shopping? If so, describe the amount and type of assistance you need.

5. Are you able to pay your bills and balance your checkbook?

Sleep and Rest

The focused interview is the most efficient way to obtain subjective information about the causes and effects of any sleep disturbances. Ask the following questions to obtain more information about a client's sleep history and patterns:

Sleep history

1. Describe any past problems you have had sleeping.

2. Do you ever fall asleep in the middle of a conversation or activity?

3. Does your spouse, family, or significant other complain that you have loud, irregular snoring?

4. Have you ever walked in your sleep? If so, describe any incidence of this behavior that you remember or what others have told you.

Sleep patterns

1. Describe what you do to prepare for bed. What do you do to make yourself sleepy?

2. What time do you go to bed? Get up?

3. How many hours of sleep do you average during the night?

4. In what position do you sleep during the night?

5. How would you describe the quality of your sleep? Restful? Restless?

6. Do you take naps during the day? If so, how long do you sleep?

7. If you are having trouble sleeping, describe the circumstances surrounding the problem. When did the problem begin? How often does it occur? Have you tried to solve the problem?

Medications, alcohol, and substance abuse

1. Are you taking any of the following drugs: hypnotics, barbiturates, sedatives, diuretics, amphetamines, or antidepressants?
2. Do you eat or drink substances with caffeine or alcohol in them?
3. Do you wake up in the morning feeling "hung over" after taking sleeping pills?
4. Do you smoke? If so, describe your smoking habits.

Illnesses

1. Have you recently gained or lost weight?
2. Do you have any illnesses that you know interfere with your sleep? If so, describe them. Diseases and conditions related to sleep disturbances include respiratory diseases, sinus problems, cardiac problems, anxiety or depression, urinary problems, arthritis or other rheumatoid disorders, hyper- or hypothyroidism, gastric ulcers, fever, liver or metabolic diseases, and migraine headaches.

Lifestyle

1. Describe in detail any recent stress or major changes in your life.
2. Would you describe your lifestyle as sedentary, moderately active, or very active?
3. Has lack of sleep affected your ability to function during the day? If so, describe how.
4. If you work, does your work schedule rotate between day and night shifts? If so, describe your work schedule over the past few months.

Nutrition

Evaluate a client's nutritional practices for intake, storage, metabolism, and use of nutrients. In addition to using a focused interview to collect information about client nutrition, you can use tools such as the 24-hour dietary recall and the dietary inventory. The following questions may help you gather information about a client's nutritional practices:

Dietary recommendations

1. How many servings of bread, rice, cereal, pasta, or other grain products do you eat each day? (Recommended: 6 to 11 servings daily)
2. How often do you eat vegetables? What kinds? (Recommended: 3 to 5 servings)
3. What types of fruit do you eat? How much? How often? (Recommended: 2 to 4 servings)
4. Do you eat dairy products like milk, yogurt, or cheese? If so, how much and how often? (Recommended: 2 to 3 servings)

5. Describe the amount of meat, fish, poultry, dried beans, eggs, and nuts you usually eat in one day. (Recommended: 2 to 3 servings)
6. Describe ways you limit the amount of fats, oils, and sweets in your diet.

General nutrition

1. Describe any recent problems you have had with eating.
2. Have you had a change in appetite recently?
3. Have you had a change in weight? If so, how many pounds? Over what period of time?
4. Have you had any recent surgery, trauma, burns, or infection?
5. How is your diet influenced by cultural or religious factors?
6. Describe your typical eating patterns. Describe what you usually eat at each meal or snack.
7. Are you on a special diet? Do you have any specific food likes or dislikes? Do you have any food allergies?
8. Do you drink alcohol? If so, how much per day or week? What kind?
9. How much coffee, tea, cola, and cocoa do you drink each day?

Food preparation

1. What facilities are available to you for meal preparation?
2. Who prepares your meals?
3. Is your income adequate to buy the food you need?

Associated behaviors

1. Do you have sores in your mouth? Do you have problems with your teeth or dentures?
2. Do you have difficulty chewing or swallowing? If so, is this associated with certain foods? With certain situations?
3. Have you had any nausea or vomiting? If so, is this associated with certain foods or situations?
4. Have you had any diarrhea or constipation? If so, for how long?
5. Do you take any prescription medications? Do you take any vitamin, mineral or nutritional supplements?
6. Have you had any surgery that may affect your nutritional status, such as an intestinal bypass?

Exercise

Use the information from a focused interview, along with clinical measures of physical fitness from the physical assessment, to determine the client's exercise habits. Ask the following questions about the client's daily exercise patterns:

Activity level

1. Describe your usual activity level: inactive, moderately active, or very active.
2. List the types of physical activity you typically engage in during the day or week.
3. Do you engage in some sort of moderate-intensity physical activity for a total of 30 minutes most days of the week?
4. Describe what you do to improve and maintain your muscle and back strength.

Safety

Clients' ability to protect themselves and prevent injury significantly contributes to a healthy lifestyle. Ask the following questions about personal safety practices:

Safety in the home

1. Describe how you maintain your home to reduce the risk of accidents to yourself and others (eg, adequate lighting, uncluttered hallways, handrails on stairs, repairs to broken windows and flooring).
2. Have you placed fire extinguishers throughout your home? Do you have a plan to exit from your home in case of fire?
3. Do you keep medications and household cleaning solutions in secure areas to reduce the risk of poisoning?
4. Describe what actions you would take if you or someone else was accidentally poisoned or became ill in your home.
5. Do you have a telephone? Are emergency phone numbers posted nearby?
6. If you live alone, does someone keep in touch with you daily?
7. If a family member or other member of your household harmed or injured you, what would you do?

Safety outside the home

1. Do you feel safe when walking alone in your neighborhood? If not, describe what you do, if anything, to protect yourself.
2. Do you live in a high-crime neighborhood or area of gang activity? If so, what do you do to keep from becoming a victim?
3. Are you able to cross streets safely when traveling on foot?
4. If you ride a bicycle, describe what you do to avoid accidents. Do you wear a bicycle helmet?

5. Do you feel safe when you take public transportation? If not, describe what steps you take to avoid being robbed, mugged, or assaulted.

6. If you drive a car, do you wear seat belts? Do you drive after you have been drinking? Do you obey the speed limit?

Safety at work

1. Do you work in what you would consider a dangerous job? If so, describe why you feel this way.

2. Describe the noise level in your work environment.

3. Are you exposed to any chemicals or environmental hazards on the job (eg, smoke, radiation, acids, or corrosive chemicals)?

4. Describe any lifting you do on the job.

5. Does your job require many repetitive motions involving your hands or wrists? If so, describe them.

6. Do you work in an extremely hot or cold environment?

7. Describe what you would do if you or someone else were injured on the job.

Family, Culture, and Environment

Environmental factors such as safety at home, in the community, and at work, and social, family, economic, religious, educational, and cultural influences can significantly affect a client's lifestyle and wellness. The best way to collect environmental data is to gather it directly from the individual, from family members, or from significant others. Use this information to identify aspects of the client's lifestyle that may need to be enhanced or supported to promote or maintain health.

Social Influences

Ask the following questions when assessing social influences on health:

1. List the members of your social network (family members, friends, peers).

2. What is the role of these individuals when you are ill?

3. What community activities are you involved in?

4. What community services are available to you? How close are you to community resources (transportation, stores, schools)?

5. Describe the neighborhood you live in.

6. Is crime a problem in your neighborhood?

Family Influences

Assess whether family attitudes and behavior regarding self-care practices are affecting the individual's health and wellness. Also assess how family members interact, depend on each other, and function as a social unit. Examine whether the family's internal and external relationships support health or are dysfunctional and, perhaps, require intervention. Assess coping styles of the family group to determine if family stress levels inhibit individual and family wellness. Ask the following questions to gather information about family influences on health:

1. Describe your family members in detail (age, sex, occupation, education).
2. How do members of the family communicate with each other?
3. Do they show interest in each others' activities? Do they listen to each other?
4. Describe how you feel your family could improve communication.
5. Have there been any major changes in the family (eg, birth of a child, loss of a job)? If so, how have family members handled these changes?
6. How are important decisions made? By one person, or by the group?
7. If one or more family members disagree, how are disputes resolved?

Economic Influences

Ask the following questions to assess economic influences on wellness:

1. Who is the main wage earner in the family?
2. Is there more than one wage earner?
3. Are there other sources of income (eg, investments, relatives)?
4. What is the total approximate income of the individual or family group? Do you feel that this amount is sufficient to meet your current and future needs?
5. Can you describe the impact your financial status has had on your standard of living, the place where you live, and your ability to stay healthy?
6. Do you feel any financial stress in your life at present (loss of job, large debt)? If so, describe it.
7. What plans have you made, if any, in case you lose part or all of your current income?

Religious Influences

The following questions may help you determine the influence religion has on your client's health:

1. Describe your religious beliefs and those of your family.
2. What role do your religious beliefs and practices play when you are healthy? Ill?

Educational Influences

Ask the following questions about a client's education level:

1. What is the primary language that you speak? Write?
2. Describe any formal schooling/education you have had.
3. Is it easier for you to learn something if you read about it? Have someone show it to you? Explain it to you?

Cultural Influences

To learn how lifestyle and health practices are influenced by the individual's cultural environment, ask the following:

1. Do you identify with any specific ethnic group? If so, which one? Do all members of your family belong to this group?
2. Describe any customs or beliefs that affect important events in your life (births, deaths, marriage, illness).
3. Do you have any cultural food preferences? Are any foods forbidden to you because of your cultural beliefs?
4. Describe why you think you get sick. Is there anything you can do to keep from getting sick? Is there anything you can do to stay healthy?

Documentation

Describe all data carefully, accurately, and objectively. You will use this information with the rest of the data you gather during the nursing health history and assessment to evaluate the client's health status and potential for supporting and promoting health. This information will help you determine the need for nursing interventions and referrals to other professionals or agencies, and will serve as a baseline for future assessments. Include aspects of the client's environment that support health as well as those that do not.

Identifying Nursing Diagnoses

After collecting information from the focused interview in each of these areas, sort the data into groups of related data or clusters of data that point to nursing diagnoses and/or collaborative problems. This will help you promote a healthy lifestyle for the client.

Chapter 4

Physical Assessment and General Survey Techniques

This chapter reviews assessment techniques for adults. Special consider-ations for infants, children, and adolescents appear in Chapter 16; for childbearing clients in Chapter 17; and for older adults in Chapter 18.

Basic Assessment Skills

The four basic assessment skills used in physical assessment are inspec-tion, palpation, percussion, and auscultation. As you apply the basic assessment skills, ask yourself the following questions:

1. What do I expect to find?
2. Are my findings *normal data, variations from the norm,* or *unexpected?*
3. How do these findings match up with other diagnostic cues?
4. Should I ask focused questions related to these findings?
5. Based on data gathered, is there anything I should pay special atten-tion to in my focused assessments of other body regions or systems?

Inspection

When inspecting, observe the client deliberately and systematically from the moment you meet the client until the end of the client-nurse interaction. Avoid the temptation to touch the client right away or use your other assessment skills first. Inspect the client in the following manner:

1. Make sure adequate daylight or strong, direct lighting is available for the inspection.
2. Survey the client's appearance.
3. Compare the client's right and left sides for symmetry.
4. Assess each body system or region, inspecting for color, texture, size, shape, contour, odor, symmetry, and movement.

5. Note any eruptions, ulcerations, or drainage.

6. For large body regions or systems, assess the entire region or system first, then each component of it.

7. Throughout the inspection, use critical thinking to determine if these findings are significant to the client's overall health.

Palpation

By touching or palpating the client with your hand, you can determine skin temperature, texture, and moisture; sense pulses, vibrations, pain, tenderness, the presence of fluid or edema, or organ distention; and determine the position, size, shape, and mobility of organs, masses, and cysts. If you notice open skin areas, sinus formations, or drainage during inspection, put on gloves. Palpate the client in the following manner:

1. To prevent discomfort, make sure your hands are warm, nails are trimmed, and jewelry is removed before starting.

2. Explain each step to client. Touch each area before palpating. Proceed slowly, with smooth, deliberate movements.

3. Use different parts of your hands for different assessments:
   - *Finger pads and palmar surface* to palpate skin texture, moisture, pulses, and superficial lymph nodes and masses
   - *Palmar aspects of fingers* to determine areas of pain and tenderness; configuration of organs and abnormal growths; presence of fluid accumulations; and body vibrations in chest and abdomen
   - *Metacarpaphalangeal joint of hand* to assess chest wall for vibrations
   - *Dorsum (back) of hand* to determine body temperature
   - *Thumb and index finger* to assess skin elasticity and skin fold thickness

4. Use different pressure, depending on the depth of the structure assessed and the thickness of tissue layers:
   - *Light palpation* is used to assess surface characteristics (eg, skin texture, a pulse, or a tender, inflamed area). Place your dominant hand perpendicular to skin with fingertips lightly touching the area being assessed, then move fingertips gently in a circular motion.
   - *Moderate palpation* is used to determine depth, size, shape, consistency, and mobility of most organs and masses and to assess any pain, tenderness, or pulsations. Place the palmar surface of your dominant hand over the structure, and press and guide fingers downward 1 to 2 cm while rotating the fingers in a circular motion.
   - *Deep palpation* is used to inspect organs or masses deep within the body cavity, or when overlying musculature is thick, tense, or rigid. Place the fingers of the nondominant hand over the fingers

of the dominant hand, and press down 2 to 4 cm. Use deep palpation with caution to avoid disseminating infections or cancerous
cells or causing underlying masses to rupture.

5. Assess a mass by placing the hands at opposite edges of mass, then
gently palpating the circumference with both hands, while visualiz-
ing mass size, shape, and depth. If it's helpful, mark the edges with
a skin-marking pen. Determine mass mobility by gently attempting
to move it slightly from side to side. Palpate the mass surface to
determine if it is smooth or irregular, noting lumps or thickened
areas. Palpate for consistency: solid (firm) or filled with fluid
(resilient).

Percussion

Percussion involves striking or tapping the body to produce sound
waves which, in turn, create tones characteristic of underlying structures. Use percussion (generally on thoracic and abdominal structures)
to determine the size and shape of organs and masses and to ascertain if
underlying tissue is solid or filled with fluid or air. Apply different
methods of percussion, depending on body area:

- *Direct percussion* to assess sinuses
- *Blunt percussion* to assess pain and tenderness in gall bladder, liver,
  and kidneys
- *Indirect percussion* for most percussion assessments

Percuss in the following manner:

1. Select the method of percussion that corresponds with body region:
   - If *direct,* tap body with fingers of one hand
   - If *blunt,* place palm of one hand flat against body and strike with
     fist of other hand
   - If *indirect,* place middle finger of nondominant hand firmly on
     area being examined keeping other fingers and palm raised.
     Position forearm of the dominant hand close to the body surface,
     with your upper arm and shoulder steady and relaxed. Swiftly
     strike middle finger on skin with the tip of middle finger of the
     dominant hand, using wrist to generate motion, then immediately
     remove striking finger. Strike with enough force to set up vibra-
     tions in body tissues, but not enough to injure the client or your-
     self. See Figure 4.1.
2. Interpret tones. The softer and shorter the tone, the more dense the
   tissue; the louder and longer the tone, the less dense the tissue.
3. Classify tones.
   - *Tympany*—loud, high-pitched, drum-like, and of medium dura-
     tion. Characteristic of organs filled with air (eg, gastric bubble in
     stomach or air-filled intestines).

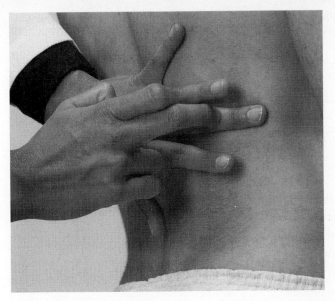

Figure 4.1   Indirect percussion.

- *Resonance*—loud, low-pitched, hollow, of long duration. Normal finding for lungs.
- *Hyperresonance*—abnormally loud, low, and of longer duration than resonance. Indicates air trapped in lungs.
- *Dullness*—high-pitched, soft, of short duration. Heard over solid organs (eg, liver).
- *Flatness*—high-pitched, softer and shorter than dullness. Occurs over solid tissue (eg, muscle and bone).
4. Repeat percussion as required, generally in systematic side-to-side or top-to-bottom manner. Note unusual sounds and complaints of pain or tenderness.

Auscultation

Auscultation is the skill of listening to the sounds produced by the body. Unassisted hearing is used to assess speech, coughing, respirations, and percussion tones. A stethoscope is used for extremely soft body sounds. When auscultating:

1. Prepare a quiet environment by turning off noisy equipment, TVs, and radios. Avoid rubbing against a client's clothes, drapes, and bedding or touching stethoscope tubing.
2. Keep the client warm because shivering obscures body sounds.

3. In addition to listening for the presence or absence of sound, listen to each sound's characteristics. Sounds may be described in terms of intensity, pitch, duration, and quality.

Equipment

Before examination, gather and organize all the equipment needed, and place it within easy reach. The following equipment is usually needed for a screening exam:

Cotton balls or wisps	Ruler (cm)
Cotton-tipped applicators	Skin-marking pen
Culture media	Slides
Dental mirror	Specimen containers
Doppler ultrasonic stethoscope	Sphygmomanometer
Flashlight	Sterile disposable needle
Gauze squares	Stethoscope
Gloves	Tape measure, flexible (cm)
Goggles	Test tubes
Lubricant	Thermometer
Nasal speculum	Tongue blade
Ophthalmoscope	Tuning fork
Otoscope	Vaginal speculum
Penlight	Vision chart
Reflex hammer	Watch with second hand

Following are some helpful hints for equipment use.

Stethoscope

- Ensure correct binaural fit: snug, comfortable, sloping forward toward nose. Use as short a section of tubing as possible (usually 12 to 18 inches).
- Wet coarse body hair on the area to be auscultated.
- Use the diaphragm for high-pitched sounds (eg, lungs and normal heart). Place the diaphragm evenly and firmly on exposed skin.
- Use the bell for low-frequency sounds (eg, heart murmurs). Place the bell lightly against the skin to form a seal, but do not flatten to diaphragm.
- Hold diaphragm/bell end against the skin with the index and middle fingers.

Doppler Ultrasonic Stethoscope

- Use for body sounds that are difficult to pick up with regular stethoscope (eg, fetal heart sounds, peripheral pulses).
- Apply a small amount of gel to the end of the Doppler probe (transducer), turn the Doppler on, and place the probe lightly against the skin over the artery to be auscultated.
- Listen for a pulsing beat.

Ophthalmoscope

- Use to inspect internal eye structures.
- Select an appropriate aperture:

  Large aperture to view dilated pupils

  Small aperture to view undilated pupils

  Red-free filter to examine the optic disc (pallor and hemorrhaging appear black)

  Grid to assess size, location, and pattern of lesions

  Slit to examine anterior eye and assess elevation/depression of lesions

- While looking through the viewing aperture, rotate lens selector to bring inner eye structures into focus, then rotate lens selection dial to adjust convergence/divergence of light: clockwise +1 to +40 for a farsighted client; counterclockwise -1 to -20 for a nearsighted client.

Otoscope

- Use to inspect internal ear structures and nose (in absence of nasal speculum).
- For an ear examination, select the largest speculum that will fit the ear canal.
- For a nose examination, select the shortest, broadest speculum that will fit the naris.

Setting Preparation

Ensure that the examination room is warm, private, and free from distractions and interruptions. It should be adequately lit (overhead lighting and a portable lamp, to highlight body surfaces and contours, are desirable) and equipped with a table or stand for examination equipment and a stool.

Position the client on the examination table (or other firm surface), situated for easy access to both sides of the client's body. Raise the table to a height that allows examination without stooping.

Client Interaction

Avoid focusing solely on the client's body. Consider the client's needs holistically.

Respect Individuality

- Individualize the physical assessment to the client's values, culture, religious beliefs, and environment.
- Explain reasons for procedures, but do not attempt to influence or coerce the client.
- Document both procedures performed and those refused.

Provide Comfort and Safety

- Show the client how to put on the examination gown, instruct the client to undress, then leave. Knock before re-entering.
- Determine if the client wishes to urinate before the examination. If urinalysis is specified, instruct the client in obtaining a clean-catch specimen.
- Wash your hands in the presence of the client.
- Anticipate the client's anxiety due to pain, embarrassment or worry, and approach gradually—first chatting, then performing familiar and non-threatening measurements such as height, weight, temperature, and pulse.
- Adapt the examination to the client's age, health status, level of functioning, and, if ill, severity of illness. To avoid exhausting the client, move around the client, don't ask the client to move.
- Anticipate potential hazards (eg, deep breathing or bending) and modify the examination as needed. Use caution with techniques that could cause injury (eg, vigorous, deep palpation).

Ensure Knowledge and Consent

- Before beginning, thoroughly explain the examination and encourage questions. (Secure a translator or someone able to use sign language, if necessary.) Have all necessary consent forms signed.
- During the examination, explain the steps in advance.
- Use the examination as an opportunity to provide client teaching.
- Inform the client if you would like another examiner to check your finding (in cases where you make an unexpected finding).

General Survey Techniques

During this initial phase of assessment, you will gather preliminary data about the client's health; assess the client's appearance, mental state, and behavior; and measure the client's height, weight, and vital signs. The general survey begins during the initial interview when you observe the client, develop initial impressions about the client's health, and formulate strategies for the examination. Use clues uncovered during the general survey to guide you during your assessment of specific body regions and systems.

General Guidelines

Position the Client

Instruct client to assume the appropriate position as required: dorsal recumbent, supine (dorsal), sitting, lithotomy, genupectoral, Sims', or prone.

Follow Universal Precautions

Hand-washing

Wash hands:

- Before and between clients
- Immediately and thoroughly with warm water and soap if you come in contact with blood, body fluids, potentially contaminated articles
- After gloves are removed
- If hand-washing facilities are not available, use a waterless, antiseptic hand cleaner.

Gloves

- Wear gloves in any situation when contact with blood and bodily fluids containing blood may occur or if you have breaks in your skin.
- Change gloves between clients.

Protective barriers

- Wear masks and protective eye wear/face shields during procedures likely to generate droplets of blood or other body fluids.
- Wear a disposable apron/gown during procedures likely to generate splatters of blood or other body fluids.

Needles and sharps

- Dispose of used needle-syringe units, scalpel blades, and other sharps in puncture-resistant containers, with needle-syringes uncapped and unbroken.
- Place puncture-resistant containers as close as is practicable to use areas.

Laundry

- Handle soiled linen as little as possible and with a minimum of agitation.
- Place linen soiled with blood or body fluids in leak-resistant bags at site of use.

Specimens

- Seal specimens of blood and body fluids in secure containers.
- When collecting specimens, avoid contaminating the outside of the container.

Blood spills

Decontaminate work surfaces after spills of blood or other body fluids with chemical germicide or 1:100 bleach-to-water solution.

Infective wastes

- Dispose of infective wastes and decontaminate material by agency policies.
- Carefully pour bulk blood, suctioned fluids, and contaminated fluids down drains connected to a sanitary sewer.

Organize the Examination

- Use a consistent pattern and routine throughout the assessment, such as head-to-toe, body systems, or a combination of the two methods.
- Perform a focused assessment on a specific organ, system, or region in response to a client complaint and before a nursing intervention or medical procedure.
- Assess by inspection, palpation, percussion, then auscultation in all body regions except the abdomen, where auscultation follows inspection.

Document Findings

Note findings throughout the exam, using standard forms if available. Document unexpected findings with complete and specific information.

Assess Appearance and Mental Status

Note any unexpected conditions of the client's appearance and mental status, taking into consideration the client's developmental stage, cultural background, socioeconomic status, job, level of intelligence, and other personal factors.

Dress and Grooming

Look at the way the client dresses for clues about the client's self-esteem and body image.

Personal Hygiene

Assess cleanliness and personal hygiene.

Gait and Posture

Confirm that the client's gait is rhythmic and free from stumbling, shuffling, and limping and that the client stands erect with shoulders level and straight.

Body Build

Check symmetry and proportions. Confirm that the arm span approximates height and that the pubis-to-crown distance roughly equals the pubis-to-sole-of-foot distance.

Behavior

Note the client's affect and mood, level of anxiety, orientation, and speech. Findings may be evaluated further during assessment of the client's psychosocial status and neurologic system.

Affect and mood

Assess the client's emotional state by noting his or her comments, body language, facial expressions, appropriateness of behavior, and comfort in talking with you.

Level of anxiety

- Observe the client for apprehension, fear, and nervousness by noting comments, body language, and facial expressions.
- If the client appears anxious, ask the client to rate his or her anxiety level on a 1 to 10 scale. Evaluate this further if no cause is found for anxiety.

Orientation

Check the client's orientation to person (knows name), place (knows location), and time (knows date and time), if he or she seems confused in the initial interview. If the client is unable to respond or responds incorrectly, perform a more detailed assessment of mental status.

Speech

- Confirm that the client speaks easily and fluently to you or an interpreter. Assess speech for quantity, volume, content, articulation, and rhythm.
- Determine if disorganized speech, silence, or constant talking indicate normal nervousness or shyness or a speech defect, neurologic deficit, depression, or other disorder.

Measure Height and Weight

Measure height and weight for baseline data, as well as to determine health. Ask the client about height and weight before measuring. Large discrepancies between assumed and actual measurements may provide clues about self image or indicate sudden loss or gain in weight due to illness. Table 4.1 lists average height and weight ranges for men and women. *Note:* Not all healthy clients will fall within these ranges.

Height

- Instruct the client to stand straight, place heels together, hold shoulders back, and look straight ahead.
- *Platform scale:* Raise the L-shaped height-attachment rod above the client's head. Extend the right-angled arm and lower it until it rests on the crown of the client's head. Read the measurement from the height-attachment rod.
- *Measuring stick attached to a wall:* Place the L-shaped level on the crown of the client's head at a right angle to the stick. Read the measurement from the stick.

Weight

- *Digital scale:* Read the weight from the display.
- *Balance-beam platform scale:* Before the client steps on, move both weights to zero and turn the knob/screw until the beam is level. After the client steps on, move the weights to the right and take a reading when the beam returns to level.
- Use a *bed scale* or a *chair scale* for clients who are unable to stand.

Measure Vital Signs

Measure vital signs to obtain baseline data, detect and monitor changes in health, and monitor clients at risk.

Body Temperature

- Use a mercury or electronic thermometer to measure oral, rectal, and axillary temperatures. Use an electronic thermometer to measure tympanic temperature.

TABLE 4.1 Metropolitan Life Insurance Company Height and Weight Tables, Men and Women, Ages 25 to 59

Height	Men Weight (lb)			Height	Women Weight (lb)		
	Small Frame	Medium Frame	Large Frame		Small Frame	Medium Frame	Large Frame
5'2"	128-134	131-141	138-150	4'10"	102-111	109-121	118-131
5'3"	130-136	133-143	140-153	4'11"	103-113	111-123	120-134
5'4"	132-138	135-145	142-156	5'0"	104-115	113-126	122-137
5'5"	134-140	137-148	144-160	5'1"	106-118	115-129	125-140
5'6"	136-142	139-151	146-164	5'2"	108-121	118-132	128-143
5'7"	138-145	142-154	149-168	5'3"	111-124	121-135	131-147
5'8"	140-148	145-157	152-172	5'4"	114-127	124-138	134-151
5'9"	142-151	148-160	155-176	5'5"	117-130	127-141	137-155
5'10"	144-154	151-163	158-180	5'6"	120-133	130-144	140-159
5'11"	146-157	154-166	161-184	5'7"	123-136	133-147	143-163
6'0"	149-160	157-170	164-188	5'8"	126-130	136-150	146-167
6'1"	152-164	160-174	168-192	5'9"	129-142	139-153	149-170
6'2"	155-168	164-178	172-197	5'10"	132-145	142-156	152-173
6'3"	158-172	167-182	176-202	5'11"	135-148	145-159	155-176
6'4"	162-176	171-187	181-207	6'0"	138-151	148-162	158-179

Mercury thermometer: Shake down to 35.5°C/96°F. Insert it in a sterile sheath (if applicable). Remove it after the proper time. Discard the sheath or wipe the thermometer toward the bulb. Hold it at eye level and rotate it until the mercury column is visible. Read the temperature scale at the upper end of the column.

Electronic thermometer: Attach a probe. Insert it in a sterile sheath. Read the temperature when it appears. Remove. Discard sheath.

- Use oral or tympanic temperature-taking methods when possible, rectal if oral is not practical, and axillary only if necessary.

Oral: Place at base of tongue in sublingual pocket to right or left of frenulum. Instruct client to keep lips closed tightly. With a mercury thermometer, leave in place for 3 to 5 minutes.

Tympanic: Accurate, least invasive, fast, and comfortable. Can only be taken with an electronic thermometer. Place covered tip of probe at ear canal opening. Activate. Read temperature. Remove. Don't force probe or occlude canal.

Rectal: Use if client is comatose, confused, or unable to close mouth. Lubricate thermometer. Put on gloves. Ask client to take a deep breath. Insert 1.5 to 4.0 cm into anus. With a mercury thermometer, leave in place for 3 minutes.

Axillary: Safest and least invasive, but least accurate. Place thermometer in client's axilla. Direct client to hold arm tightly across chest. With a mercury thermometer, leave in place for 9 minutes.

Pulse

- Palpate the radial pulse by placing the pads of the first three fingers on anterior wrist along the radius bone.
- Assess pulse rate, rhythm, force, and elasticity.

Rate: Regular pulse rate: count for 30 seconds and multiply by 2. Irregular pulse rate: count for 1 minute.

Rhythm: Confirm that intervals between beats are constant.

Force: Note pressure required before the pulse is felt.

Elasticity: Palpate along the artery proximal to distal, to confirm that the artery feels smooth, straight, and resilient.

Respirations

For even breathing, count the number of breaths for 30 seconds and multiply by 2; for irregular or difficult breathing, count for 1 minute. To help the client maintain a normal respiratory rate, assume the posture for counting the radial pulse while counting breaths.

Blood Pressure

- Before measuring, ensure that the client is comfortable and has been at rest for at least 5 minutes.
- Select the proper pressure cuff size. (Take measurements in the arm if possible, thigh or leg if not.)
- *For an arm blood pressure measurement:* Remove clothing from the arm and place the cuff on the arm smoothly and snugly, with its lower border 1 inch above the antecubital area. Slightly flex the arm and hold it at heart level with the palm up. Place the bell-shaped diaphragm of the stethoscope over the brachial pulse. Pump up the cuff until the sphygmomanometer registers 30 mm Hg above the point at which the brachial pulse disappears. Release the valve on the cuff so that pressure decreases at 2 to 3 mm Hg/sec; note the manometer reading at the 5 phases (Korotkoff's sounds). Deflate the cuff rapidly and remove it.

Summary of General Survey Techniques

General Guidelines

1. Position client.
2. Follow universal precautions.
3. Organize the examination.
4. Document findings.

Assess Appearance and Mental Status

1. Dress and grooming
2. Personal hygiene
3. Gait and posture
4. Body build
5. Behavior

Measure Height and Weight

Measure Vital Signs

1. Body temperature
2. Pulse
3. Respirations
4. Blood pressure

Chapter 5

Assessing the Integumentary System

Focused Interview

The appearance of the skin can have considerable impact on self-image because many people perceive themselves in relation to how they believe they appear to others. During your focused assessment of the integumentary system, you will be asking about a client's lifestyle, self-care, relationships with others, health patterns and problems, and methods of coping with skin problems. Be especially considerate of how you investigate a client with a skin disorder.

Skin and Glands

1. Describe your skin today; 2 months ago; 2 years ago. Have you ever had a skin problem? If so, please describe it and any treatment or resolution.

2. Is there a history of allergies, rashes, or other skin problems in your family? Have you noticed any rashes on your body? Do you have any skin pain or discomfort? Do you have any sores or ulcers on your body that are slow in healing? Where? Do you have frequent boils or skin infections? If so, please describe (where it started, where it spread, when you first noticed it, when it occurs, if you've traveled recently).

3. How do you care for your skin? What kind of skin cleaning products do you use? How often do you bathe? How often do you clean your clothes? Do you have trouble controlling body odor? How much and how easily do you sweat?

4. Have you had an illness recently? Are you taking any medications?

5. How would you describe your level of stress? Has it changed recently?

6. Have you noticed any changes in the color of your skin?

7. Does your skin itch? If so, where? How severe is it? Describe the environment in which it occurs.

8. Have you noticed any changes in the size, color, shape, or appearance of any moles or birthmarks? Any pain, itching, or bleeding? If so, when did you first notice the change?

9. Does your job or hobby require you to work with any chemicals? Do you need to wear a specific type of protective equipment?

10. Has the condition of your skin affected your relationships in any way? Has it limited you in any way? If so, how?

Hair

1. Describe your hair now; 2 months ago; 2 years ago. Have you ever had problems with your hair? If so, please describe the problem, including any treatment and resolution.

2. How often do you wash your hair? Do you have excessive dandruff; if so, how do you try to control it?

3. Have you noticed increased hair loss recently? If so, describe how the hair fell out. Any illnesses in the last few months? Are you taking any medications (including oral contraceptives) or receiving chemotherapy?

4. How do you style your hair? Please describe any styling products and equipment (blow dryer, curling iron, etc.) used. Do you frequently set your hair in corn-rows or tight braids? Do you bleach, color, perm, or chemically straighten your hair? If so, how often?

5. Do you pluck your eyebrows or facial hair? Do you shave or otherwise remove the hair on your face, legs, or under your arms?

6. Do you swim regularly?

Nails

1. Describe your nails now; 2 months ago; 2 years ago. Have you ever had problems with your nails? If so, please describe the problem, including any treatment and resolution.

2. Have you noticed any pain, swelling or drainage around your cuticles? When did you first notice it? What do you think might have caused it?

3. Have you been ill recently? Are you taking any medications?

4. Do you wear nail polish or artificial nails?

5. Do you spend a great deal of time at work or at home with your hands in water?

Physical Assessment

- Gather the following equipment:

centimeter ruler	examination light
drape	magnifying glass
examination gloves	penlight
examination gown	Wood's lamp

- Put on gloves if you notice open skin areas, sinus formations, or drainage.

Assessment Techniques/ Normal Findings	Special Considerations

Skin

1. Position the client.
Have client sit, wearing only an examination gown and drape.

2. Confirm that skin is clean and free from body odor.
If client has just come from work or has another reason not to be clean, body odor may be present.

Increased urea and ammonia may occur in clients with kidney disorders.

3. Observe skin tone.
- Evaluate widespread color changes such as pallor, cyanosis, erythema, or jaundice.
- Assess cyanotic clients for vital signs and level of consciousness.

Pallor or cyanosis indicates abnormally low plasma oxygen, placing client at risk for altered tissue perfusion.

Alert!
Be alert for possibility of shock if pallor is accompanied by drop in blood pressure, increased pulse and respirations, and marked anxiety. If these cues are present, consult a physician immediately.

4. Inspect skin for even pigmentation.
Confirm normal pigmentation variations and normal appearance of freckles and nevi.

Clients with vitiligo may have a severely disturbed body image.

Assessment Techniques/ Normal Findings	Special Considerations
5. Determine skin temperature. • Using dorsal surface of hand, palpate forehead or face, then palpate inferiorly, including hands and feet, comparing temperature on right and left sides. • Verify normal temperatures— mildly cool to slightly warm— and similar temperatures on either side.	Skin temperature is higher than normal with systemic infections or with metabolic disorders such as hyperthyroidism, after vigorous activity, and when external environment is warm. One side warmer than normal may indicate inflammation on that side. Skin temperature is lower than normal with metabolic disorders such as hypothyroidism or when external environment is cool. Localized coolness results from decreased circulation due to vasoconstriction or occlusion, which may occur from peripheral arterial insufficiency. Bilateral temperature difference may indicate an interruption or lack of circulation on the cool side due to compression, immobilization, or elevation.
6. Assess amount of moisture on skin. Inspect and palpate face, skin folds, axillae, palms, and soles of feet. Skin with a fine sheen of perspiration and/or oil and moderately dry skin are not abnormal.	*Diaphoresis* occurs during exertion, fever, pain, emotional stress, and with metabolic disorders such as hyperthyroidism. Diaphoresis also may indicate an impending medical crisis such as a myocardial infarction. *Pruritus,* which frequently accompanies dry skin, may lead to abrasion and thickening. Localized itchiness may indicate a skin allergy.

Assessment Techniques/ Normal Findings	Special Considerations
	Generalized dryness may occur with dehydration or hypothyroidism. Dry, parched lips and mucous membranes of the mouth are indicators of systemic dehydration. Dry skin over lower legs may indicate vascular insufficiency.
7. Palpate skin for texture. Use palmar surface of fingers and finger pads to confirm smooth, firm, and even skin.	Skin may become excessively smooth and velvety with hyperthyroidism, rough and scaly with hypothyroidism.
8. Palpate skin to determine thickness. Verify that outer layer of skin is thin and firm over most of the body; thicker over palms, soles, elbows, and knees; and thinner over eyelids and lips.	Very thin, shiny skin may occur with impaired circulation.
9. Palpate skin for elasticity. • With forefinger and thumb, grasp and then release a fold of skin beneath clavicle or on radial aspect of wrist. Verify that skin is mobile and resilient.	Tenting, resulting from decreased turgor, occurs with dehydration or after substantial weight loss. Increased skin turgor may be caused by scleroderma, in which underlying connective tissue becomes scarred and immobile.
• Firmly palpate the feet, ankles, and sacrum. Edema is present if palpation leaves a dent. • Grade edema from 1 (mild) to 4 (deep). See Figure 5.1.	Edema makes the skin look puffy, pitted, and tight, and is most noticeable on feet, ankles, and in sacral area.

Assessment Techniques/ Normal Findings	Special Considerations

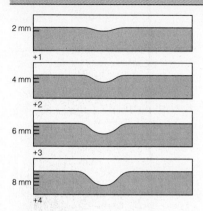

2 mm

+1

4 mm

+2

6 mm

+3

8 mm

+4

Figure 5.1 Four-point scale for grading edema.

10. Inspect skin for superficial arteries and veins.
A fine network of veins or a few dilated blood vessels visible just beneath surface where skin is thin (eg, abdomen and eyelids) is normal.

11. Inspect and palpate skin for lesions.
- Carefully inspect client's body, including skin folds and crevices. *Primary lesions* develop on previously unaltered skin. *Secondary lesions* are lesions that change over time or because of scratching, abrasion, or infection. Freckles, insect bites, healed scars, and certain birthmarks are normal lesions.

Widespread lesions may indicate systemic or genetic disorders or allergic reactions. Localized lesions may indicate physical trauma, chemical irritants, or allergic dermatitis.

Tables 5.1 and 5.2 (pp. 47-49) describe and classify primary and secondary lesions, respectively.

Assessment Techniques/ Normal Findings	Special Considerations

Alert!

Put on gloves if you notice drainage from any lesions.

- Palpate lesions between thumb and index finger. Measure all lesion dimensions, including height (cm), if possible.
- Document lesion size (cm).
- Shine Wood's light on skin to distinguish fluorescing lesions.
- Assess any drainage for color, odor, consistency, amount, and location. If indicated, obtain specimen of drainage for culture and sensitivity.

Observe periumbilical and flank areas for *ecchymosis* (bruising). Ecchymosis in periumbilical area may signal bleeding in abdomen. Ecchymoses in flank area are associated with pancreatitis or bleeding in the peritoneum.

Referral

If you suspect physical abuse, obtain medical assistance and follow your state's legal requirements to notify the police or local protective agency. Some signs of abuse include bruises or welts in a pattern, burns with sharply demarcated edges, additional injuries such as fractures and dislocations, and multiple injuries in various stages of healing. Be especially sensitive if client is fearful of family members, is reluctant to return home, or has a history of previous injuries.

Referral

If you see track marks and suspect substance abuse, refer client to mental health or substance abuse professional.

12. Palpate skin for sensitivity.

Alert!

Localized hot, red, swollen, or painful areas indicate inflammation and possible infection. Do not palpate.

Palpate skin and skin lesions in various regions of the body and ask client to describe sensations as closely as possible. Document findings, especially pain or discomfort. Client should not report any discomfort.

TABLE 5.1 Primary Skin Lesions

Macule, Patch

Flat, nonpalpable change in skin color. Macules are smaller than 1 cm with a circumscribed border, and patches are larger than 1 cm and may have an irregular border.

Examples: Macules: freckles, measles, and petechiae. Patches: mongolian spots, port-wine stains, vitiligo, and chloasma.

Papule, Plaque

Elevated, solid, palpable mass with circumscribed border. Papules are smaller than 0.5 cm; plaques are groups of papules that form lesions larger than 0.5 cm.

Examples: Papules: elevated moles, warts, and lichen planus. Plaques: psoriasis, actinic keratosis, and also lichen planus.

Nodule, Tumor

Elevated, solid, hard or soft palpable mass extending deeper into the dermis than a papule. Nodules have circumscribed borders and are 0.5 to 2 cm; tumors may have irregular borders and are larger than 2 cm.

Examples: Nodules: small lipoma, squamous cell carcinoma, fibroma, and intradermal nevi. Tumors: large lipoma, carcinoma, and hemangioma.

Vesicle, Bulla

Elevated, fluid-filled, round or oval shaped, palpable mass with thin, translucent walls and circumscribed borders. Vesicles are smaller than 0.5 cm; bullae are larger than 0.5 cm.

Examples: Vesicles: herpes simplex/zoster, early chickenpox, poison ivy, and small burn blisters. Bullae: contact dermatitis, friction blisters, and large burn blisters.

Wheal

Elevated, often reddish area with irregular border caused by diffuse fluid in tissues rather than free fluid in a cavity, as in vesicles. Size varies.

Examples: Insect bites and hives (extensive wheals).

(continued)

TABLE 5.1 Primary Skin Lesions *(continued)*

Pustule

Elevated, pus-filled vesicle or bulla with circumscribed border. Size varies.

Examples: Acne, impetigo, and carbuncles (large boils).

Cyst

Elevated, encapsulated, fluid-filled or semisolid mass originating in the subcutaneous tissue or dermis, usually 1 cm or larger.

Examples: Varieties include sebaceous cysts and epidermoid cysts.

TABLE 5.2 Secondary Skin Lesions

Atrophy

A translucent, dry, paperlike, sometimes wrinkled skin surface resulting from thinning or wasting of the skin due to loss of collagen and elastin.

Examples: Striae, aged skin.

Erosion

Wearing away of the superficial epidermis causing a moist, shallow depression. Beause erosions do not extend into the dermis, they heal without scarring.

Examples: Scratch marks, ruptured vesicles.

Lichenification

Rough, thickened, hardened area of epidermis resulting from chronic irritation such as scratching or rubbing.

Examples: Chronic dermatitis.

(continued)

TABLE 5.2   Secondary Skin Lesions (continued)

Scales

Shedding flakes of greasy, keratinized skin tissue. Color may be white, gray, or silver. Texture may vary from fine to thick.

Examples: Dry skin, dandruff, psoriasis, and eczema.

Crust

Dry blood, serum, or pus left on the skin surface when vesicles or pustules burst. Can be red-brown, orange, or yellow. Large crusts that adhere to the skin surface are called scabs.

Examples: Eczema, impetigo, herpes, or scabs following abrasion.

Ulcer

Deep, irregularly shaped area of skin loss extending into the dermis or subcutaneous tissue. May bleed. May leave scar.

Examples: Decubitus ulcers (pressure sores), stasis ulcers, chancres.

Fissure

Linear crack with sharp edges, extending into the dermis.

Examples: Cracks at the corners of the mouth or in the hands, athlete's foot.

Scar

Flat, irregular area of connective tissue left after a lesion or wound has healed. New scars may be red or purple; older scars may be silvery or white.

Examples: Healed surgical wound or injury, healed acne.

Keloid

Elevated, irregular, darkened area of excess scar tissue caused by excessive collagen formation during healing. Extends beyond the site of the original injury. Higher incidence in people of African descent.

Examples: Keloid from ear-piercing or surgery.

Assessment Techniques/ Normal Findings	Special Considerations

Scalp and Hair

1. Confirm that scalp and hair are clean.
Ask client to remove any hair accessories. Part and divide hair at one-inch intervals and observe.

Excessive dandruff occurs with skin disorders such as psoriasis.

Distinguish dandruff from head lice.

2. Observe hair color.

Graying in patches may indicate a nutritional deficiency (commonly of protein or copper).

3. Assess hair texture.
• Roll a few hair strands between thumb and forefinger.
• Hold a few hair strands taut, then slide thumb and forefinger along length of strands.

Metabolic disorders such as hypothyroidism, as well as nutritional deficiencies, may result in dull, dry, brittle, and coarse hair.

4. Observe amount and distribution of hair.
Confirm that hair distribution is even. Remember to assess amount, texture, and distribution of body hair.

In most people, hair growth declines by age 50. Widespread hair loss may be caused by illness, infections, metabolic disorders, nutritional deficiencies, and chemotherapy. Patchy hair loss may be due to infection.

Male pattern baldness is the most frequent cause of hair loss in men, but has no clinical significance.

5. Inspect scalp for lesions.
• Dim room light and shine Wood's lamp on scalp while parting hair.
• Confirm that scalp is free from lesions and areas of fluorescent glow.
• Check scalp for excoriation from itching.

Gray, scaly patches with broken hair may indicate a fungal infection, such as ringworm.

Areas that fluoresce indicate infection.

Head lice usually cause intense itching.

Assessment Techniques/ Normal Findings	Special Considerations

Nails

1. Confirm that nails are clean and well groomed.

Dirty fingernails may indicate a self-care deficit, but could also be related to a person's occupation.

2. Inspect nails for even, pink undertone.
Small, white markings are normal.

Nails appear pale and colorless with peripheral arteriosclerosis or anemia, yellow with jaundice, and dark red with polycythemia. Fungus infections may cause nails to discolor. Horizontal white bands may occur in chronic hepatic or renal disease.

Referral
A darkly pigmented band in a single nail may indicate melanoma in nail matrix. Refer to a physician.

3. Assess capillary refill.
Depress nail edge briefly to blanch, then release. Color returns instantly to healthy nails.

Nail beds appear blue and color return is sluggish with cardiovascular or respiratory disorders.

4. Inspect and palpate nails for shape and contour.
- Perform Schamroth technique to assess clubbing.
- Ask client to bring the dorsal aspect of corresponding fingers together, creating a mirror image.
- Look at distal phalanx and observe diamond-shaped opening created by nails; if clubbing is present, diamond is not formed (Figure 5.2).

Fingernail clubbing occurs with hypoxia or prolonged impaired peripheral tissue perfusion, as well as with cirrhosis, colitis, or thyroid disease. Ends of fingers become enlarged, soft, and spongy, and nail angle exceeds 160 degrees (Figure 5.3).

Assessment Techniques/ Normal Findings	Special Considerations

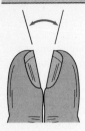

Figure 5.2 Schamroth technique.

Nails normally form a slight convex curve or lie flat. Confirm normal 160-degree angle between skin and nail base (Figure 5.4).

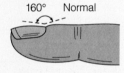

Figure 5.4 Normal nail.

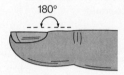

Figure 5.3 Clubbing of the nail.

Spoon nails, which form a concave curve, are associated with iron deficiency. (Figure 5.5).

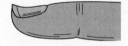

Figure 5.5 Spoon nail.

5. Palpate nails to determine thickness, regularity, and attachment to nail bed.
Confirm normal characteristics: smooth, strong, and regular; firmly attached to nail bed; and only slightly mobile.

Thickened nails may indicate circulatory disorders. Onycholysis occurs with trauma, infection, and skin lesions.

6. Inspect and palpate cuticles.
Confirm that cuticles are smooth and flat.

Untreated hang nails can become inflamed and lead to paronychia.

Nursing Diagnoses Commonly Associated with the Integumentary System

- **Impaired tissue integrity**—damaged or destroyed tissue
- **Impaired skin integrity**—disrupted skin surface, destroyed skin layers, and invaded body structures

Common Integumentary System Alterations

Contact dermatitis, herpes simplex, eczema, herpes zoster, impetigo, basal cell carcinoma, psoriasis, squamous cell carcinoma, tinea, malignant melanoma, measles, Kaposi's sarcoma, German measles, hirsutism, chickenpox, paronychia.

Integumentary System Client Education

Stress the importance of the following guidelines for maintaining healthy skin and preventing future skin problems.

Skin and Glands

- *Dry skin:* Wash morning and night with mild soap. Apply lotion with sunscreen daily. Apply lotion after bathing if excessively dry.
- *Oily skin*: Wash two to three times daily with warm washcloth and glycerine soap. Avoid fatted soap, oils, lotions, and creams.
- Prevent hair sprays and other hair products from touching face.
- Avoid contact with chemicals and contaminants by use of protective clothing and safety equipment. Do not use personal care products, soaps, detergents, food, clothing, jewelry, etc., that cause skin irritation.
- Do not try to tan. Use sunscreen of at least SPF 15. Wear protective hats and clothing. Know skin cancer risk factors and self-assessment procedures.
- Do not smoke.
- Get regular exercise.

Hair and Nails

- Avoid frequent chemical styling procedures. Refrain from vigorous brushing, combing, teasing, and picking. Avoid tight braiding or corn rowing.
- Do not share brushes, combs, and other implements.
- Keep toenails trimmed. Wear shoes with room for toes to move.

Integumentary System Physical Assessment Summary

Skin and Glands

1. Position the client.
2. Confirm that skin is clean and free from body odor.
3. Observe skin tone.
4. Inspect skin for even pigmentation.
5. Determine skin temperature.
6. Assess amount of moisture on skin.
7. Palpate skin for texture.
8. Palpate skin to determine thickness.
9. Palpate skin for elasticity.
10. Inspect skin for superficial arteries and veins.
11. Inspect and palpate skin for lesions.
12. Palpate skin for sensitivity.

Scalp and Hair

1. Confirm that scalp and hair are clean.
2. Observe hair color.
3. Assess hair texture.
4. Observe amount and distribution of hair.
5. Inspect scalp for lesions.

Nails

1. Confirm that nails are clean and well groomed.
2. Inspect nails for even, pink undertone.
3. Assess capillary refill.
4. Inspect and palpate nails for shape and contour.
5. Palpate nails to determine thickness, regularity, and attachment to nail bed.
6. Inspect and palpate cuticles.

Chapter 6

Assessing the Head and Neck

Focused Interview

Prior to the interview, be sure to review any diagnostic test results, including X-rays, CT scans, MRI studies, hearing and sight tests, and blood studies, to identify what additional information you need to obtain from the assessment. If the client presents a problem of the head or neck, or if there is a family history of a problem in this area, obtain a thorough history of each complaint. Matters related to the respiratory, gastrointestinal, neurological, and musculoskeletal systems may apply.

Head

1. Do you have headaches? If so, please describe frequency, onset, duration, location, character, associated symptoms, precipitating factors, and treatment.
2. Have you had any dizziness, loss of consciousness, seizures, or blurred vision? If so, when, for how long, and what did you do to relieve the symptom?
3. Have you noticed any swelling, lumps, bumps, or skin sores on your head that did not heal?
4. Describe any recent injury you have had to your head. How did it occur? Did you lose consciousness (for how long)? Did you have symptoms afterwards? How and where were you treated?

Eyes

1. Have you noticed any recent changes to your vision? Have you had to take measures to compensate for the loss?
2. When was your last eye examination? What were the results?

3. Do you wear glasses or contact lenses? Please describe vision with and without them. How long do you wear your contact lenses? How do you clean and care for them?

4. Have you ever experienced blurred vision, double vision, sensitivity to light, burning, or itching? Do you ever see small black spots that seem to move when you are looking at something? Do you ever see halos around lights?

5. Have you had any eye pain?

6. Have you ever had any eye injury or eye surgery?

7. Have you or any family member had diabetes, hypertension, or glaucoma?

8. Do you have trouble seeing at night?

9. What kinds of activities do you perform at work? What are your hobbies?

Ears

1. Have you noticed any change in your hearing? If so, describe onset, character, and situations of loss.

2. Has any member of your family had ear problems or hearing loss?

3. When was your last hearing test? What were the results? Does your hearing seem better in one ear than the other? Do you own or use a hearing aid?

4. Are you frequently exposed to loud noise? When? How often? For how long? Are protective devices available and do you use them?

5. Do you have any pain in your ears? Describe it.

6. Have you had any ear drainage? Describe it.

7. Have you had ringing in your ears, dizziness, nausea, or vomiting?

8. Do you experience ear infections or irritations after swimming or being exposed to dust or smoke?

9. Are you taking any medications?

10. How do you clean your ears?

Nose and Sinuses

1. Are you having problems with your nose or sinuses? If so, describe them. Are you able to breathe through your nose? Can you breathe through both nostrils?

2. Do you have nasal discharge? If so, is it continuous or occasional?

3. Do you have nosebleeds? How often? How do you treat them? What is your usual blood pressure? Do you use nasal sprays?

4. Have you ever had a nose injury or nose surgery? Describe it and the treatment. Do you have any residual problems as a result?

5. Describe your sense of smell.

6. What medications do you take to relieve your nasal symptoms? What other drugs (prescribed, over-the-counter, illicit) do you take?

Mouth and Throat

1. How would you describe the condition of your mouth and teeth? Any changes in the last few months?
2. Do you have problems swallowing?
3. Do you have any sores or lesions in your mouth or on your tongue? Describe. Are they present constantly or do they come and go periodically?
4. How often do you brush? Floss? Do your gums bleed frequently?
5. What dental problems, surgery, or procedures have you had? Do you wear dentures, partial plates, retainers, or any other removable or permanent appliance? Why do you wear it? Does it fit comfortably and well?
6. When was your last dental examination? Are there any foods you are unable to eat because of problems with your teeth? Do you have pain in one or more of your teeth?
7. Do you have frequent sore throats? Have you noticed any hoarseness or loss of voice?
8. Have you ever smoked or chewed tobacco or dipped snuff? How much? How often?

Neck

1. Have you noticed any lumps or swelling on your neck?
2. Has your neck been weak, sore, or stiff?
3. Have you ever had any thyroid gland problem? If so, have you had thyroid surgery and are you taking thyroid medication?

Physical Assessment

- Gather the following equipment:

cotton-tipped applicator	ophthalmoscope
cover card	otoscope
examination gloves	penlight
examination gown	Snellen's or Tumble E chart
gauze square	sterile cotton balls
Jaeger card	tongue depressors
nasal speculum	tuning fork

- Put on gloves before examining eyes, nose, mouth, and any areas with open skin or drainage.

Assessment Techniques/ Normal Findings	Special Considerations

Head

1. Position the client.
Have client sit comfortably on
examination table.

2. Inspect head and scalp.
- Note size, shape, symmetry, and
  integrity. Identify frontal, pari-
  etal, and occipital prominences.
- Confirm that eyes, ears, nose,
  and mouth are symmetrical.

**3. Observe movements of head,
face, and eyes.**

Jerky movements or tics may
result from neurologic or psychologic disorders.

4. Palpate head and scalp.
Note contour, size, and texture.
Ask client to report any tender-
ness during palpation.

Note any tenderness, swelling,
edema, or masses which require
further evaluation.

**5. Confirm skin and tissue
integrity.**

Alert!
Put on gloves if you notice any open
area or drainage. Examine drainage
for color, odor, consistency, amount,
and location. If indicated, obtain a
specimen for lab analysis.

Note any alteration in skin or tissue integrity related to ulcerations, rashes, discolorations, or
swelling.

6. Palpate temporal artery.
Palpate between eye and top of ear
to check smoothness.

Thickening or tenderness could
indicate inflammation.

7. Auscultate temporal artery.

A swishing sound (bruit) may
indicate a cardiac or vascular
problem.

Assessment Techniques/ Normal Findings	Special Considerations

8. Test range of motion of temporomandibular joint.
Place fingers in front of each ear and have client slowly open and close mouth. Slight joint indentation is normal.

Limitation of movement or tenderness upon movement indicates need for further evaluation.

Eyes

1. Test distant vision.
- Clients who wear corrective lenses should be tested first with the lenses and then without.
- Ensure that room is well lit and eye chart is at proper height. Position client exactly 20 feet from chart. Ask client to cover one eye with card and read smallest line of letters possible. Repeat with other eye, then with both eyes uncovered. Record numbers at end of last line read.
- Observe client's behavior while reading chart. Verify that client reads English.

Referral
If vision is poorer than 20/30 and uncorrected, refer client to an ophthalmologist.

Frowning, leaning forward, and squinting indicate reading difficulty.

2. Test near vision.
Have client hold Jaeger card 14 inches from eyes. Ask client to cover one eye with cover card and read. Repeat test with other eye, then with both eyes uncovered. Record results.

Inability to see objects at close range is called hyperopia. In persons over 45, it is called presbyopia.

Referral
If client is unable to read letters at 14 inches, refer to ophthalmologist.

3. Test visual fields by confrontation.
- This test assumes examiner has normal peripheral vision.

Assessment Techniques/ Normal Findings	Special Considerations

- Stand 2 to 3 feet in front of client at eye level. Ask client to cover one eye with card while you cover your opposite eye. Holding penlight equidistant between client and you, extend arm upward, then move it from periphery to midline point.
- Ask client to report when object is first seen. Repeat procedure upward, toward the nose, and downward. Repeat entire procedure with other eye covered.

Inability of client to see penlight when examiner does could indicate peripheral vision loss and necessitates further evaluation.

4. Test six cardinal fields of gaze.

- Stand about 2 feet in front of client. Ask client to hold head steady while following the penlight with eyes.
- Starting in midline, move penlight through the six cardinal fields of gaze as shown in Figure 6.1.
- Assess client's ability to follow movements. If client moves head, hold chin steady with free hand.

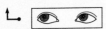

1. Penlight is to nurse's extreme left.

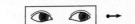

4. Penlight is to nurse's extreme right.

2. Penlight is left and up.

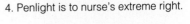

5. Penlight is right and up.

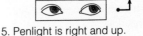

3. Penlight is left and down.

6. Penlight is right and down.

Figure 6.1 Testing the six cardinal fields of gaze.

Assessment Techniques/ Normal Findings	Special Considerations

5. Assess corneal light reflex.

- Ask client to stare straight ahead as you shine penlight about 12 inches from eyes.
- Check that reflection in pupils appears in same spot.

Asymmetrical reflection may indicate extraocular muscle weakness.

6. Perform cover test.

- Ask client to stare straight ahead at a fixed point.
- Cover one eye with card and determine if uncovered eye remains focused on designated point.
- Remove card and confirm that previously covered eye remains focused straight ahead.

Movement of either eye may indicate eye muscle weakness.

- Repeat with other eye.

7. Inspect pupils.

Confirm that pupils are round, equal in size and shape, and in center of eye.

8. Evaluate pupillary response.

- Dim lights so pupils dilate.
- Ask client to stare straight ahead.
- Move penlight in from client's side and shine directly into one eye.
- Observe whether illuminated and unilluminated pupil constrict simultaneously.

Failure of illuminated pupil to constrict indicates defect in direct pupillary response. Failure of unilluminated pupil to constrict indicates defect in consensual response. Failure of both pupils to constrict indicates problem in pupillary response controlled by cranial nerves II (optic) and III (oculomotor).

Assessment Techniques/ Normal Findings	Special Considerations

9. Test accommodation of pupils.
- Ask client to stare straight ahead at a distant point.
- Hold penlight 4 to 5 inches from client's nose, then ask client to shift gaze from distant point to penlight.
- Confirm that eyes converge and pupils constrict as eyes focus.

10. Record client's response to tests.
Record normal response as PER-RLA: Pupils Equal, Round, React to Light and Accommodation.

11. Inspect external eye.
- Stand directly in front of client. Confirm that eyelids symmetrically cover eyeballs when closed, eyebrows are symmetrical, eyelashes are similar in quantity and distribution, and eyeball is neither protruding nor sunken.
- Shine penlight from side across each cornea and confirm that each is clear with no irregularities.

Ptosis can be caused by a dysfunction of cranial nerve III (oculomotor). Eyes protruding beyond supraorbital ridge can indicate thyroid disorder. However, this trait may be normal for client.

12. Examine conjunctiva and sclera.
For each eye, gently separate eyelids and ask client to look up, down, and to each side. Assess for healthy characteristics: moist and clear conjunctiva with small blood vessels, clear lens, white sclera, and round iris of the same color.

Eyelid edema can be caused by allergies, heart disease, or kidney disease. Inability to move eyelids can indicate dysfunction of nervous system.

Inflammation and edema of conjunctiva indicate infection or possible foreign body.

Assessment Techniques/ Normal Findings	Special Considerations

13. Inspect inner eye with oph- thalmoscope.

- Dim lights. Ask client to look at a fixed point straight ahead.
- To examine client's right eye, hold instrument in right hand over your right eye. Stand at a slight angle lateral to the client's line of vision.
- Place your left hand on client's shoulder or forehead. Hold opthalmoscope against your head, directing the light into the client's pupil. Keep your other eye open. Approach client at a 15-degree angle toward the nose.
- As you look into the client's pupil, locate the red reflex. If necessary, adjust lens wheel to focus. In a normal eye, no shad- ows or dots will interrupt red reflex.
- Keep advancing toward the client until opthalmoscope is almost touching client's eye- lashes. Focus on ocular fundus (Figure 6.2). Locate optic disc (normally a round or oval yel- low-orange depression with a distinct margin), macula, and fovea centralis.

Persistent absence of red reflex may indicate a cataract.

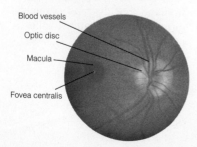

Blood vessels
Optic disc
Macula
Fovea centralis

Figure 6.2   The optic disc.

Assessment Techniques/ Normal Findings	Special Considerations

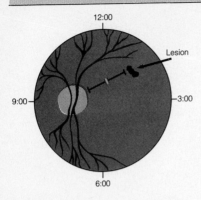

Figure 6.3 Documenting a finding from the opthalmoscopic exam.

- Systematically inspect structures. A scleral crescent or pigment crescent around the margin of the optic disc is normal. Document any findings using the optic disc as a clock face and the diameter of the disc for noting its distance from the optic disc (Figure 6.3).

Degeneration of macula—which may be due to hemorrhages, cysts or other alterations—is common in older adults and results in impaired central vision. Abnormalities of retinal structures appear as dark or opaque spots on the retina, an irregularly-shaped optic disc, lesions, or hemorrhages on the fundus.

- Trace the path of a paired artery and vein from the optic disc to the periphery in each quadrant. Note number, color, and width of major blood vessels and any crossing of blood vessels.
- Repeat entire procedure for left eye using your left hand and left eye.

Absence of major vessels in any quadrant is abnormal. Constricted arteries appear less than 2/3 the diameter of accompanying veins. Vessels crossing more than 2 DD from the optic disc and extremely tortuous vessels require further evaluation.

Ears

1. Inspect external ear for symmetry, proportion, color, and integrity.

Assessment Techniques/ Normal Findings	Special Considerations
Confirm that external auditory meatus is patent, with no drainage. Check that ear color matches surrounding skin and face, without redness, nodules, swelling, or lesions.	Discharge, redness, or swelling may indicate infection or allergy.
2. Palpate auricle and push on tragus. Confirm absence of hard nodules, lesions, swelling, and pain. The tragus should be moveable.	Hard nodules are a sign of gout. Pain could result from an infection of the external ear or temporo-mandibular joint dysfunction with pressure on tragus. Lesions accompanied by a history of long-term sun exposure may be cancerous.
3. Palpate mastoid process lying directly behind ear. Check for lesions, swelling, and pain.	Abnormal finding could indicate mastoiditis.
4. Inspect auditory canal using otoscope. • Ask client to tilt head away from you toward opposite shoulder. Hold otoscope between palm and first two fingers of one hand, with handle up or down. • Stabilize the head and straighten the canal with your other hand. (Pull the pinna up, back, and out to straighten.) • With the light on, insert speculum into ear. Confirm that external canal is open and free from tenderness, inflammation,	Cerumen occluding ear canal must be removed.

Assessment Techniques/ Normal Findings	Special Considerations

lesions, growths, discharge, and foreign substances. Note amount, texture, and color of cerumen.

Alert!
Use care when inserting speculum into ear. Avoid pressing speculum against sides of auditory canal.

5. Examine tympanic membrane using otoscope.

- Observe membrane for normal conditions: flat, gray, intact, and no scars.
- Confirm cone-shaped reflection of otoscope light at 5 o'clock in right ear and 7 o'clock in left. Look for shadow of the short process of the malleus behind tympanic membrane. Membrane should be intact.
- If you cannot visualize the tympanic membrance, remove the otoscope, reposition the auricle and reinsert the otoscope. Do not reposition auricle with otoscope in place.

White patches on tympanic membrane indicate prior infections. Yellow or reddish tympanic membrane could indicate middle-ear infection. Bulging tympanic membrane may indicate increased pressure in middle ear; retracted tympanic membrane may indicate vacuum in middle ear.

6. Assess tympanic membrane using otoscope during Valsalva maneuver.
With tympanic membrane in clear view, ask client to close lips, pinch nose, and gently blow nose. Confirm that tympanic membrane flutters toward otoscope slightly.

Rigidity of tympanic membrane, which could be due to variety of alterations, requires further evaluation.

Alert!
Do not ask clients who are elderly or who have upper respiratory infections to perform the Valsalva maneuver.

Assessment Techniques/ Normal Findings	Special Considerations
7. Perform whisper test. Ask client to hold heel of hand over one ear. Cover your mouth so client cannot see your lips. Standing 1 to 2 feet from client, whisper a simple phrase. Ask client to repeat phrase. Repeat for other ear.	Inability to repeat phrase may indicate loss of ability to hear high-frequency sounds.
8. Perform Rinne test. • Gently strike tuning fork on palm of hand to start vibrating. Place base of fork on client's mastoid process. • Ask client to tell you when sound is no longer heard. Note number of seconds. • Immediately move tines of still-vibrating fork in 1 to 2 cm in front of external auditory meatus, and ask client to tell you when sound is no longer heard. Note number of seconds. • Tuning fork sound normally carries twice as long by air conduction as by bone.	Hearing bone-conducted sound as long as or longer than air-conducted sound indicates possibility of conductive hearing loss.
9. Perform Weber test. • Place base of vibrating tuning fork against skull (midline of anterior portion of frontal bone or midline of forehead). • Ask client if sound is heard equally or better in one ear. If equal, record as "no lateralization" (normal). If one side is better, ask which and record as "sound lateralizes to [right or left] ear."	Unequal hearing may be due to poor conduction or to nerve damage. With poor conduction, sound will be heard better in impaired ear; with nerve damage, sound will be referred to stronger ear.

Assessment Techniques/ Normal Findings	Special Considerations

Nose and Sinuses

1. Inspect nose for symmetry, shape, skin lesions, and signs of infection.

Discharge or noisy breathing may indicate obstruction or infection.

2. Test for patency.
Press finger on one nostril. Confirm that client can breathe freely through opposite side. Repeat with other nostril.

Inability to breathe through each naris could indicate severe inflammation or obstruction.

3. Inspect nasal cavity using nasal speculum.
- Stabilize client's head with non-dominant hand. Insert speculum with blades closed into naris. Then separate blades, dilating naris. Avoid hitting septum.
- With client's head erect, inspect inferior turbinates. With client's head tilted back, inspect middle meatus and middle turbinates.
- Confirm that mucosa is dark pink and smooth, without swelling, discharge, bleeding, or foreign bodies. Confirm that septum is midline, straight, and intact. Repeat on other side.

Swollen and red mucosa may indicate upper respiratory infection. Swollen and pale mucosa or nasal polyps may indicate chronic allergies. A deviated septum appears as an irregular lump in one nasal cavity. (Slight deviations generally are not problems.) A perforated septum may permit light to shine from one naris into the other.

4. Palpate sinuses.
Press thumbs over frontal sinuses below eyebrows, then over maxillary sinuses below cheekbones.

Tenderness upon palpation may indicate chronic allergies or sinusitis.

Assessment Techniques/ Normal Findings	Special Considerations

Mouth and Throat

Alert!
Put on gloves before proceeding
with the following assessments.

1. Inspect and palpate lips.
Confirm that lips are symmetrical,
smooth, pink, moist, and without
lesions.

Lesions or blisters may be caused
by herpes simplex virus; lesions
must be evaluated for cancer.
Pallor of lips may indicate
cyanosis.

2. Inspect teeth.
Observe client's dental hygiene.
Ask client to clench teeth and
smile while you observe occlusion. Confirm that teeth are white,
smooth, and free of debris.

Loose, painful, broken, and mis-
aligned teeth, malocclusion, and
inflamed gums need further evaluation.

**3. Inspect and palpate buccal
mucosa, gums, and tongue.**
• Look into client's mouth under
strong light. Confirm that
tongue is pink and moist, with
papillae on dorsal surface.

Smooth, coated, or hairy tongue is
usually related to dehydration or
disease. A small tongue may indicate undernutrition.

• Ask client to touch roof of
mouth with tip of tongue.
Ventral surface should be
smooth and pink.

Tongue tremor may indicate dysfunction of cranial nerve XII
(hypoglossal) nerve.

• Palpate area under tongue.
Using gauze pad, grasp tongue
and inspect for lesions, lumps,
and nodules. Confirm that tissue is smooth.

Persistent lesions on tongue
require further evaluation—particularly lesions on sides or at base
of tongue.

• Hold tongue aside with tongue
depressor while inspecting
mucous lining of mouth and
gums. Confirm that lining is
pink, moist, smooth, and free of
lesions.
• Confirm integrity of soft and
hard palates.

Gums that are bleeding, retracted,
or overgrown onto teeth are dis-
eased.

Assessment Techniques/ Normal Findings	Special Considerations

4. Inspect salivary glands.
Locate all salivary ducts and assess for pain, tenderness, swelling, and redness.

5. Inspect throat.
- Use tongue depressor and penlight to examine throat. Ask client to open mouth wide, tilt head back, and say "aah." Confirm that uvula rises in midline.
- Depress middle of arched tongue with tongue depressor to clearly examine throat while client says "aah." Check that soft palate rises.
- Observe tonsils (if not removed), uvula, and posterior pharynx for normal characteristics: pink, with no inflammation, swelling, or lesions. Confirm slight vascularity of tonsils.
- Note mouth odors.

Viral pharyngitis may accompany a cold. Tonsils may be bright red, swollen, and may have white spots on them.

Sweet, fruity breath indicates diabetic acidosis; ammonia odor indicates kidney disease.

Neck

1. Inspect neck for skin color, integrity, shape, and symmetry.
Check for swelling of lymph nodes below jaw angle and along sternocleidomastoid. Confirm that head is held erect, with no tremors.

Excessive rigidity of neck may indicate arthritis, while inability to hold neck still may be due to muscle spasms. Swelling of lymph nodes, which may indicate infection, requires further assessment (see Step 8 on p. 72).

2. Test range of motion of neck.
Alert!
Assess range of motion of neck slowly to prevent dizziness.

Assessment Techniques/ Normal Findings	Special Considerations
Ask client to drop chin to chest, turn head right and left, touch left ear to left shoulder and right ear to right shoulder (without raising shoulders), then extend head back. Ask client to report any pain while you note any limitation of movement.	Pain or limitation of movement could indicate arthritis, muscle spasm, or inflammation.
3. Observe carotid arteries and jugular vein.	Distention or prominence may indicate vascular disorder.
4. Palpate trachea. Place thumb and index finger on each side of trachea just above sternal notch. Lightly palpate. Confirm that trachea is midline and equidistant to sternocleido-mastoid muscle and that hyoid bone and tracheal cartilages move when client swallows.	Tracheal displacement results from masses in the neck or medi-astinum; pneumothorax; and fibrosis.
5. Inspect thyroid gland. Assess size and shape of thyroid. To help distinguish thyroid from other neck structures, ask client to take a sip of water. Adjust lighting to cast shadows as needed.	Enlargement of thyroid and mass-es near the thyroid appear as bulges during swallowing.
6. Palpate thyroid gland from behind client. • Give client a cup of water to hold. Stand behind client. Ask client to sit up straight. • For right side, ask client to lower chin, and turn head slightly to right. With left hand, push trachea to right. With right hand, palpate area between tra-chea and sternocleidomastoid.	An enlarged thyroid gland may be due to a metabolic disorder such as hyperthyroidism. Document the location, size, and shape of palpable masses 5 mm and larger and evaluate client further.

Assessment Techniques/ Normal Findings	Special Considerations

Slowly and gently retract sternocleidomastoid, then ask client to take a sip of water. Palpate as thyroid gland moves up during swallowing.

• Reverse procedure for left side.

Alert!
Never attempt to palpate both lobes of the thyroid simultaneously.

7. Auscultate thyroid.
If thyroid is enlarged, auscultate area to detect any bruits.

Bruits are abnormal and indicate increased blood flow.

8. Palpate head and neck lymph nodes.

• Ask client to bend head toward side being examined. Palpate lymph nodes by exerting gentle pressure with fingertips of both hands on the node groups. Figure 6.4 illustrates a suggested sequence for palpation.

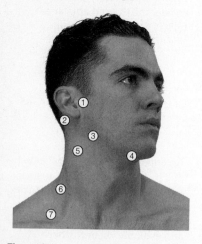

Figure 6.4 Suggested sequence for palpating lymph nodes.

Assessment Techniques/ Normal Findings	Special Considerations
• Document location, size, shape, fixation or mobility, and tenderness of any palpable lymph nodes.	Lymphadenopathy can result from infection, allergies, or tumor.

Nursing Diagnoses Commonly Associated with the Head and Neck Region

- **Sensory/perceptual alteration: visual, auditory, olfactory**—a change in the amount or interpretation of incoming stimuli accompanied by absent, diminished, exaggerated, or distorted response to such stimuli; not a result of mental or personality disorders
- **Impaired swallowing**—decreased ability to voluntarily pass fluids and/or solids from mouth to stomach
- **Altered oral mucous membrane**—disruptions in tissue layers of oral cavity
- **Impaired home maintenance management**—inability to maintain safe home environment due to alteration in vision or hearing
- **Body image disturbance**
- **Ineffective individual coping**
- **High risk for injury**
- **Acute or chronic pain**
- **Powerlessness**

Common Head and Neck Region Alterations

Head and Neck

Acromegaly, Bell's palsy, Cushing's syndrome, Down syndrome, fetal alcohol syndrome, headaches, hydrocephalus, hyperthyroidism, torticollis.

Eyes

Arcus senilis, cataract, chalazion, conjunctivitis, diabetic retinopathy, ectropion, entropion, exophthalmos, glaucoma, hordeolum, pterygium, ptosis, strabismus.

Ears

Hemotympanum, otitis externa, otitis media, perforation of tympanic membrane, scarred tympanic membrane, tophi, tympanostomy tubes.

Nose and Sinuses

Deviated septum, epistaxis, nasal polyps, perforated septum, rhinitis, sinusitis.

Mouth and Throat

Ankyloglossia, aphthous ulcers, black hairy tongue, gingival hyperplasia, gingivitis, leukoplakia, carcinoma, herpes simplex, tonsillitis, smooth tongue.

Head and Neck Region Client Education

All clients need information on health promotion and self-monitoring for the head and neck region. Provide information about the care of chronic disease as appropriate, as well as the following:

Head and Neck

- Recognize cancer warning signs: unexplained lumps or thickening; changes in size or color of warts or moles; difficulty in swallowing, unusual bleeding or discharge; sores that do not heal; and persistent hoarseness or cough.
- Wear protective head gear for potentially dangerous work, recreation, and other activities.
- Learn relaxation techniques to help deal with chronic headaches and jaw or neck pain.

Eyes

- Have eyes examined every 5 years if under age 40; every 2 years if over age 40. Undergo glaucoma screening every 2 years if over age 40; 1 year if over age 65, particularly if you have a family history of glaucoma or eye injury.
- Wear protective eyewear for potentially dangerous work, recreation, and other activities. Wear ultraviolet-B absorbent dark glasses in sun.
- Know signs of eye diseases such as excessive tearing, diplopia, halo around lights, reduced field of vision, flashes of light, dimming or distortion of vision, photophobia, night blindness, change in color vision, and pain.
- Do not rub itching or burning eyes. Use plain white tissue (without dyes) if eyes are chronically dry.
- *Vision impaired:* learn about social service agencies and training and financial assistance. Maintain a consistent and clutter-free environ-

ment. Determine availability of options to enhance daily living (eg, books on tape, animal companions).

- *Contact lens wearers:* know possible signs of keratitis—abnormal sensitivity to light, reduced vision, halos around objects, and acute pain. Disinfect daily. Do not swim with lenses.

Ears

- Never put objects into ear canal (including cotton swabs). Clean external ear with soft cloth and mild soap.
- *Hearing impaired:* understand need for, use of, and care of hearing aids and other devices to enhance hearing and safety (eg, lights on telephones, closed-caption TV). Advise client's family and friends to speak to client in normal tones.
- If you have an upper respiratory infection with heavy nasal discharge, remember to blow nose gently, to avoid possible ear infection.
- Wear hearing protection when around loud music, aircraft, explosives, firearms, and other loud noises. Screen hearing of children and elderly adults annually.

Nose and Sinuses

- Know proper use and side effects of prescription medications and nasal sprays.
- Learn how to care for nosebleeds. Monitor blood pressure if nosebleeds are frequent.

Mouth and Throat

- Brush teeth, use dental floss, and clean oral appliances correctly.
- Do not smoke or use smokeless tobacco.
- Have teeth examined yearly.

Head and Neck Region Physical Assessment Summary

Head

1. Position the client.
2. Inspect head and scalp.
3. Observe movements of head, face, and eyes.
4. Palpate head and scalp.
5. Confirm skin and tissue integrity.
6. Palpate temporal artery.
7. Auscultate temporal artery.
8. Test range of motion of temporomandibular joint.

Eyes

1. Test distant vision.
2. Test near vision.
3. Test visual fields by confrontation.
4. Test six cardinal fields of gaze.
5. Assess corneal light reflex.
6. Perform cover test.
7. Inspect pupils.
8. Evaluate pupillary response.
9. Test accommodation of pupils.
10. Record client's response to tests.
11. Inspect external eye.
12. Examine conjunctiva and sclera.
13. Inspect inner eye with ophthalmoscope.

Ears

1. Inspect external ear for symmetry, proportion, color, and integrity.
2. Palpate auricle and push on tragus.
3. Palpate mastoid process lying directly behind ear.
4. Inspect auditory canal using otoscope.
5. Examine tympanic membrane using otoscope.
6. Assess tympanic membrane using otoscope during Valsalva maneuver.
7. Perform whisper test.
8. Perform Rinne test.
9. Perform Weber test.

Nose and Sinuses

1. Inspect nose for symmetry, shape, skin lesions, and signs of infection.
2. Test for patency.
3. Inspect nasal cavity using nasal speculum.
4. Palpate sinuses.

Mouth and Throat

1. Inspect and palpate lips.
2. Inspect teeth.
3. Inspect and palpate buccal mucosa, gums, and tongue.
4. Inspect salivary glands.
5. Inspect throat.

Neck

1. Inspect neck for skin color, integrity, shape, and symmetry.
2. Test range of motion of neck.
3. Observe carotid arteries and jugular vein.
4. Palpate trachea.
5. Inspect thyroid gland.
6. Palpate thyroid gland from behind client.
7. Auscultate thyroid.
8. Palpate head and neck lymph nodes.

Chapter 7

Assessing the Respiratory System

Focused Interview

Review results of chest X-rays, scans and tomography, blood studies, pulmonary-function tests, and any other relevant diagnostic work before conducting the focused interview. Before beginning the interview, determine the present respiratory status of the client. Postpone a detailed interview if the client demonstrates dyspnea, cyanosis, difficulty with speech and accompanying anxiety.

Question client about respiratory patterns, respiratory problems, and lifestyle and environmental conditions that might affect the respiratory system. Consider client's developmental stage, psychosocial factors, and self-care factors.

Respiratory System

1. Do you have any problems breathing now? In the past? When you are having problems, what makes your breathing easier? Worse? Do you use a nebulizer, oxygen, humidifier, or other device to help improve your breathing? Does your breathing problem stop you from doing a specific task? Does the breathing problem make you dizzy, light-headed, or confused?

2. Do you smoke? What? When did you start? How much in 24 hours? Have you ever tried to stop smoking? If so, what happened? Do you live with a smoker?

3. Do you have a cough? If so, how often does it occur? What do you think causes it? Is it worse at any time of day or night? Describe the cough (dry, hacking, hoarse, barking, or wet). Do you cough up sputum? If so, please describe look, odor, amount, color, and consistency and any recent changes. Do you have trouble coughing up sputum? Does coughing hurt? If so, describe type, severity, and location of

pain and what you do to ease the pain. Does your coughing awaken you at night or make you tired? How do you stop coughing? Ask for name, dose, and frequency of any medications.

4. Do you live or work in an environment that exposes you to caustic fumes, fungi, or other known carcinogens? Do you work in a dust-producing environment? If so, do you wear any protective devices to keep your lungs clean?

5. Do you have frequent colds? Have you had a respiratory infection in the last 2 years? If so, when and what were the symptoms and treatment?

6. Does anyone in your family have respiratory disorders, including inherited or genetic disorders affecting respiratory function?

7. Do you experience itching, running nose and eyes, or other allergic symptoms? Do you have pets? Are you allergic to fur, feathers, or dander? If so, how do you react? Have you been tested for allergies? If so, what were the results?

8. Have you lost or gained weight recently? If so, how much in what time period?

9. Have you recently traveled to a rural area or foreign country?

Physical Assessment

Gather the following equipment:

drape	face mask
examination gloves	metric ruler
examination gown	skin marker
examination light	stethoscope

Assessment Techniques/ Normal Findings	Special Considerations

Alert!

Put on gloves before examining eyes, nose, mouth, and any areas with open skin or drainage. Use universal precautions if client is coughing or sneezing.

Assessment Techniques/ Normal Findings	Special Considerations

Survey

1. Survey client.

Make rapid survey to determine client's ability to participate in exam. Inspect client's appearance and position. Confirm that respiration is effortless; facial color is consistent with body; expression is relaxed; client is breathing through nose, with lips closed without circumoral pallor; right and left chest movement is equal; and no supraclavicular or intercostal retractions are noted.

Clients with any degree of dyspnea will be unable to participate in the assessment. Note inability to sit up unassisted, labored breathing, and altered consciousness.

Referral

Clients experiencing dyspnea who are restless, anxious, and unable to follow directions may need immediate medical assistance.

Thorax Inspection

1. Position client.

Have client sit with all clothing removed to waist except exam gown and drape.

2. Count respirations for 1 minute.

- Observe rate, rhythm, and depth of respiratory cycle.
- Observe chest movement in anterior, posterior, and lateral thorax.
- Confirm that respirations— about 12 to 18 per minute—are quiet, symmetrical, and effortless.
- Ask client to take deep breath while you observe muscular involvement.

Males tend to breathe abdominally, females more costally, and male and female athletes and singers abdominally.

Table 7.1 describes altered respiratory patterns.

Table 7.1   Altered Respiratory Patterns

Type	Pattern	Common Causes
Tachypnea	Rate faster than 24 per minute	Anxiety, pain, or reduced chest expansion caused by enlarged abdominal organs, respiratory insufficiency, pneumonia, pleurisy, and alkalosis
Bradypnea	Rate less than 12 per minute	Upper abdominal or chest pain, electrolyte imbalance, or neurologic damage
Hyperpnea (hyperventilation)	Rapid and deep breathing	Anxiety, exercise, or neurologic or metabolic disease
Kussmaul's respirations	Very deep respirations	Metabolic acidosis
Cheyne-Stokes respirations	Respirations with alternating cycles of deep, rapid breathing followed by periods of apnea	Occur during sleep or with approaching death
Sighing	Frequent sighing	Lack of oxygen or air hunger
Ataxic breathing (Biot's respirations)	Varying depth and rate followed by periods of apnea	Disease of respiratory centers of the brain
Air trapping	Overexpansion of chest and rapid, shallow respirations	Chronic obstructive lung disease: increased bronchial resistance during expiration traps air

Assessment Techniques/ Normal Findings	Special Considerations
3. Inspect skin color. Confirm that chest wall skin color is consistent with that of the rest of the body.	Evaluate further if pallor, cyanosis, or a flushed ruddy color is evident.
4. Inspect configuration of chest. Confirm that the transverse diameter:anteroposterior diameter ratio is about 2:1.	Evaluate further with ratio deviation.
5. Determine thorax symmetry. Standing behind client, draw imaginary line across superior border of scapulae from right to left acromion and confirm that the line is perpendicular to the vertebral line.	Uneven scapulae could indicate a pneumonectomy as well as scoliosis or kyphosis.

Posterior Thorax Palpation

1. Lightly palpate posterior aspect of chest.

- Assess muscle mass and area directly below skin for masses. Palpate chest using finger pads, including areas superior to scapulae, below 12th rib, and laterally to midaxillary lines.
- Confirm that muscle mass is firm and that skin and subcutaneous area are free of masses, lesions, and pain.

Painful areas over posterior thorax may indicate inflamed fibrous connective tissue. Painful areas overlying intercostal spaces suggest inflamed pleura. Crepitus occurs when air escapes into subcutaneous tissue.

2. Palpate posterior thorax for respiratory expansion.

- Place hands about level with the 8th to 10th ribs, with thumbs close to vertebral line. Gently press skin between thumbs, keeping palms in contact with client.

Assessment Techniques/ Normal Findings	Special Considerations
• Ask client to take a deep breath. Confirm that you feel equal pressure on your hands, and that your thumbs move evenly away from vertebral line.	Decreased chest expansion could indicate neuromuscular or tracheobronchial disease. Decrease on only one side may result from a lung, pleural, or skeletal problem.
3. Palpate posterior thorax for tactile fremitus. Palpate areas shown in Figure 7.1 with metacarpophalangeal joint area or ulnar surface of your hand while client repeatedly says "99" or "1-2-3." Note <u>fremitus</u>.	Diminished vibrations over trachea or bronchi area may result because client needs to speak louder, but also could indicate tracheobronchial tree obstruction. Lung consolidation increases vibrations.

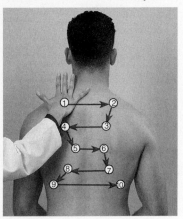

fremitus is the vibration felt on the outer chest wall as the client speaks. "99"

Figure 7.1 Palpating for tactile fremitus.

Posterior Thorax Percussion

1. Position client.
Help client lean slightly forward and round shoulders.

Assessment Techniques/ Normal Findings	Special Considerations

2. Percuss lungs.

- Percuss over apex of left lung, then over apex of right lung.
- Systematically percuss each intercostal space to lowest rib and extending to left and right midaxillary lines in the order shown in Figure 7.2. (Do not percuss over vertebrae, scapulae, or ribs.)
- Confirm resonant sound over lungs.

Hyperresonant sound suggests possible pneumothorax, but could be normal in elderly clients.

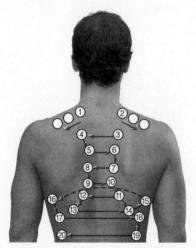

Figure 7.2   Pattern for percussing posterior thorax.

3. Percuss to determine excursion of diaphragm.

- Beginning at 7th intercostal space, percuss downward along a scapular line to level of diaphragm. Confirm that resonance changes to dullness. Mark skin.

Assessment Techniques/ Normal Findings	Special Considerations
• Ask client to take a deep breath and hold it. Percuss downward from skin mark to dull sound. Mark skin.	
• Ask client to take several normal breaths, then take one normal breath and exhale as much as possible and hold breath. Percuss upward until you hear resonance. Mark skin. Have client breathe normally. • Repeat on other scapular line. • Have client relax.	Shortened posterior excursion indicates inability or unwillingness to take full breath due to pain, anxiety, abdominal pressure, or phrenic nerve damage. Client with posterior excursion shorter than 3 cm is not breathing effectively and may not be exchanging gases or perfusing tissue adequately.

Posterior Thorax Auscultation

1. Auscultate posterior thorax.

• Ask client to slowly breathe in and out of mouth. Place diaphragm of stethoscope firmly on chest wall. • Auscultate from vertebral line at C7 to T3. Confirm that sound is bronchial. Table 7.2 lists normal breath sounds.	Do not confuse static-like sounds from chest hair or fabric with breath sounds.

Alert!
Monitor breathing to prevent hyperventilation.

• Move stethoscope to right and left of vertebral line at T4 to T5 level. Confirm that sound is bronchovesicular.	Diminished or absent sound may indicate obstruction from masses, mucous plugs, or foreign object.
• Systematically auscultate over apices of lungs, each intercostal space to lowest rib, and extending to left and right midaxillary lines in the order shown in Figure 7.3. Confirm that sound is vesicular.	Clients with emphysema produce diminished lung sounds. Bronchial or bronchovesicular sounds usually indicate lung-tissue consolidation.

Table 7.2 Normal Breath Sounds

Type	Description	Location	Characteristics
Vesicular	Soft-intensity, low-pitched, "gentle sighing" sounds created by air moving through smaller airways (bronchioles and alveoli)	Over peripheral lung; best heard at base of lungs	Best heard on inspiration, which is about 2.5 times longer than the expiratory phase (5:2 ratio)
Bronchovesicular	Moderate-intensity and moderate-pitched "blowing" sounds created by air moving through larger airways (bronchi)	Between the scapulae and lateral to the sternum at the first and second intercostal spaces	Equal inspiratory and expiratory phases (1:1 ratio)
Bronchial (tubular)	High-pitched, loud, "harsh" sounds created by air moving through the trachea	Anteriorly over the trachea; not normally heard over lung tissue	Louder than vesicular sounds; have a short inspiratory phase and long expiratory phase (1:2 ratio)

Source: B Kozier, G Erb, and R Olivieri, *Fundamentals of Nursing*, 5th ed. (Redwood City, CA.: Addison-Wesley Nursing, 1995), p. 403.

Assessment Techniques/ Normal Findings	Special Considerations

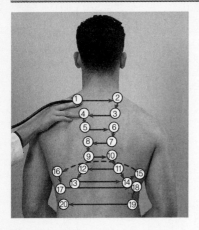

Figure 7.3 Pattern for auscultating posterior thorax.

2. Listen for adventitious sounds. Note location, quality, duration, and occurrence.

Table 7.3 describes adventitious sounds.

Anterior Thorax Percussion

1. Percuss anterior thorax.

- Systematically percuss, beginning at apices and continuing to diaphragm level, making sure finger is in intercostal space parallel to ribs. Extend to midaxillary line on each side as shown in Figure 7.4. (Avoid percussing over sternum, clavicle, ribs, and heart.)
- Have female clients move breasts if necessary.

Alert!
Be sensitive to client's privacy; limit exposure of body parts.

Table 7.3 Adventitious Sounds

Sound	Characteristics	Occurrence
Crackles or rales	A series of popping noises similar to a "frying" sound heard in the chest as air coming in suddenly opens the small deflated air passages that are coated and sticky with exudate	Inspiration
Coarse rales	Loud, crackling, moist sounds that are low-pitched and bubbling	Inspiration Possible expiration
Medium rales	Similar to but not as loud as coarse rales	Middle of inspiration
Fine rales	Noncontinuous popping sound that is high-pitched, short, and crackling	End of inspiration
Rhonchi (sonorous wheeze)	Continuous, low-pitched, prolonged, deep, and rumbling sound caused by passage of air through trachea or bronchi obstructed by secretions, spasm, or growth	More pronounced during expiration
Wheezes (sibilant rhonchi)	Continuous, high-pitched, musical sound caused by air forced through narrowed respiratory passages	Inspiration and expiration Louder during expiration
Pleural friction rub	Low-pitched, dry, grating sound caused by the rubbing of two inflamed pleural surfaces	Inspiration and expiration

Assessment Techniques/ Normal Findings	Special Considerations

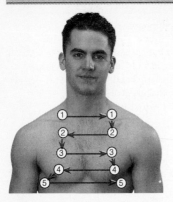

Figure 7.4 Pattern for percussing and auscultating anterior thorax.

Anterior Thorax Auscultation

1. Auscultate anterior thorax.

- Confirm that sound is bronchial over trachea; bronchovesicular over right and left primary bronchi; and vesicular over lung parenchyma (Figure 7.5).
- Note location, quality, and occurrence of any adventitious sounds.

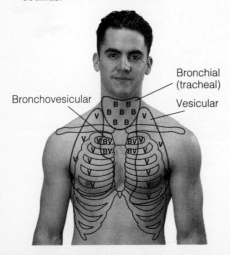

Figure 7.5 Auscultatory sounds

Nursing Diagnoses Commonly Associated with the Respiratory System

- **Ineffective airway clearance**—inability to clear secretions or obstructions from respiratory tract to maintain airway patency
- **Ineffective breathing pattern**—inhalation and/or exhalation pattern that does not enable adequate pulmonary inflation or emptying
- **Impaired gas exchange**—decreased passage of oxygen and/or carbon dioxide between alveoli of lungs and vascular system

Common Respiratory System Alterations

Atelectasis, asthma, bronchitis, emphysema, pneumonia, pneumothorax.

Respiratory System Client Education

Discuss general care, risk factors, and preventive health care of the respiratory system.

General Respiratory System Care

- Smoking is the primary risk factor for lung cancer. If you smoke, quit. Try to maintain a smoke-free home and workplace.
- Exercise daily. *If asthmatic:* focus on swimming and activities requiring short bursts of energy, and avoid cold-weather and nonstop activities. Pretreat with albuterol and theophylline, if necessary.
- Consider yearly influenza immunization.
- Use precautions when with large groups of people and when with person experiencing upper respiratory infection.
- Avoid pollutants, allergens, and other contaminants. Keep the home free from dust and other allergic irritants. Vacuum regularly. Consider removing pets from home if allergic to them. Eliminate ragweed and wild grasses from yards.
- Use a humidifier or dehumidifier appropriately.
- Change filters in air conditioners and heaters regularly.
- Use face masks and other protective equipment.
- Avoid anxiety, stress, and fatigue, which may worsen symptoms of respiratory problems.

Respiratory System Physical Assessment Summary

Survey

1. Survey client.

Thorax Inspection

1. Position client.
2. Count respirations for 1 minute.
3. Inspect skin color.
4. Inspect configuration of chest.
5. Determine thorax symmetry.

Posterior Thorax Palpation

1. Lightly palpate posterior aspect of chest.
2. Palpate posterior thorax for respiratory expansion.
3. Palpate posterior thorax for tactile fremitus.

Posterior Thorax Percussion

1. Position client.
2. Percuss lungs.
3. Percuss to determine excursion of diaphragm.

Posterior Thorax Auscultation

1. Auscultate posterior thorax.
2. Listen for adventitious sounds

Anterior Thorax Percussion

1. Percuss anterior thorax.

Anterior Thorax Auscultation

1. Auscultate anterior thorax.

Chapter 8

Assessing the Cardiovascular System

Focused Interview

Question client about the status and extent of his or her wellness and knowledge about maintaining optimal cardiovascular health.

Level of Wellness

1. How do you feel? Can you physically and mentally perform all the activities necessary to meet your personal and work-related needs?
2. Do you exercise? What is the frequency, intensity, duration, and mode? What is your understanding about the benefits and type of exercise selected?
3. Do you monitor pulse and blood pressure? When? How often? Demonstrate how you monitor and describe the type of blood pressure monitor you use. What are your readings?
4. What types of food do you eat, how often, and how much? Do you keep track of fat, protein, and carbohydrate intake? Do you know the difference between saturated and unsaturated fat? How much fiber do you consume? Do you add salt and other flavor enhancers to food? If so, what, how much, and how often? Do you diet? If so, describe type, duration, supplementation, and if it is medically supervised. Do you take vitamins, protein supplements, or antioxidants? What is your nonalcoholic fluid intake?
5. What is your weight? Have you gained or lost weight recently? If so, over how much time? Do you know your percentage of body fat? Are you retaining fluid? If so, when did it start and has retention been progressing slowly or rapidly accelerating?
6. What is your present occupation? How many hours do you work in a typical week? Do you work on weekends? What do you do to unwind? How would you describe your personality? What are the major stressors in your life? What do you do to manage stress?

7. Do you smoke? If so, what, for how long, and how much? Are you frequently exposed to passive smoke? If so, where and for how long?

8. Do you take cocaine, alcohol, or other illicit drugs? If so, describe type, amount, frequency, and duration of use.

9. Do you fear developing cardiovascular disease?

10. Have you been tested recently for cardiovascular wellness? If so, what were the tests, how long ago, and what were the results?

Risk for Developing Cardiovascular Disease

1. Has any family member ever had cardiovascular disease or symptoms commonly associated with it?

2. Do you have a history of cardiovascular disease? If so, what disease, when did it develop, and what were the symptoms? How old were you? How was it treated? Were the interventions repeated?

3. Have you ever had a history of medical conditions such as diabetes, neurologic disorders, recent dental work (or past dental complications), thyroid disorders, or venereal disease?

4. Determine client's risk factor profile for developing cardiovascular disease based on the following: heredity, sex, race, age, smoking, hypertension, elevated total cholesterol/LDL/triglycerides, diabetes, high body fat composition, sedentary lifestyle, excessive stress, diet rich in saturated fats, and Type A personality.

Ability to Modify Risk Factors

1. Do you know the risk factors for developing cardiovascular disease?

2. Do you know which risk factors you have some control over? State how you think you can realistically modify these risk factors.

Presence and Management of Cardiovascular Disease

1. Have you experienced symptoms that may suggest the presence of cardiovascular disease: activity intolerance, anorexia, bloody sputum, changes in sexual practices, confusion or alterations in mental status, chest discomfort, coughing, dizziness, dyspnea, fatigue, fever, hoarseness, frequent night-time urination, leg pains after activity, sleeping pattern alteration, syncope, palpitation, or swelling? If so, describe in detail.

2. Can you identify precipitating factors for the symptoms?

3. What is the quality of the symptom: sharp, dull, pressure-like, piercing, or ripping?

4. Where is the symptom located? Does the symptom radiate to other parts of the body? What relieves the symptom? What is the severity

of the symptom(s)—from 1 (hardly noticeable) to 10 (worst discomfort ever experienced)? What is the timing of the symptom? Predictable? What is the duration of the symptom—constant, or does it wax and wane? Are symptoms isolated or in combination?

5. If you have any symptoms, have you seen a doctor about them? What is being done for them? Are you taking cardiac medications? If so, what, how often, what dose, what frequency, and with what side effects?

6. What do you do to maintain your health in the presence of cardiovascular disease?

Women's Cardiovascular Wellness and Risk for Disease

1. Are you menstruating? If not, at what age did menopause begin? Did you have a hysterectomy? Were your ovaries removed?

2. Do you take oral contraceptives?

Physical Assessment

Gather the following equipment:

appropriate lighting	drape	two metric rulers
Doppler (optional)	stethoscope	

Assessment Techniques/ Normal Findings	Special Considerations

Inspection

1. Position client.
Begin with client seated upright with chest undraped.

2. Inspect face.
- Assess facial skin color for uniformity.
- Evaluate general appearance of face for relative uniformity and flatness.

Note the following skin conditions and disease associations: flushed skin and rheumatic heart disease or fever; grayish undertones and coronary artery disease or shock; a ruddy color and polycythemia or Cushing's syndrome.

Assessment Techniques/ Normal Findings	Special Considerations

3. Inspect eyes.
Examine eyes and periorbital areas:

- Confirm eye uniformity and absence of protruding appearance.

Protruding eyes are seen in hyperthyroidism.

- Verify that periorbital areas are relatively flat, without puffiness.

Puffiness may result from fluid retention, myxedema, or valvular heart disease.

- Confirm whitish color of sclera and absence of arcus in corneas.

Blue color in sclera is associated with Marfan's syndrome.

An arcus in a young person may indicate hypercholesteremia. In persons of African descent it may be normal.

- Confirm pinkish color of conjunctiva.
- Check eyelids for smoothness.

Xanthelasmas indicate premature atherosclerosis.

4. Inspect lips.
Confirm uniform color without underlying tinge of blue.

Blue-tinged lips may indicate cyanosis.

5. Inspect earlobes.
Confirm that earlobes are relatively smooth without creases (unless injured).

Bilateral earlobe creases are often associated with coronary artery disease, especially in young adults (Figure 8.1).

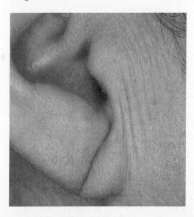

Figure 8.1 Ear lobe crease.

Assessment Techniques/ Normal Findings	Special Considerations

6. Inspect head.

- Observe ability of client to hold head steady.

Head bobbing up and down in synchrony with heartbeat is characteristic of severe aortic regurgitation.

- Assess structure of skull and proportion of skull to face.

A protruding skull is found with Paget's disease.

7. Inspect jugular veins.

- With client sitting upright with head turned slightly away, use lamp to cast shadows on neck. Look for external and internal jugular veins over and under sternocleidomastoid muscle (not normally visible in upright sitting position).

- If you can visualize the jugular veins, measure their distance superior to clavicle. If jugular vein pulsations are visible, palpate radial pulse and determine if pulsations coincide with pulse.

Jugular vein pulsations that are obvious, are present during inspiration and expiration, and coincide with arterial pulse are commonly seen with severe congestive heart failure.

- Have client lie at a 45-degree angle (if client can tolerate this position without pain and can breathe comfortably). Place a ruler vertically at the angle of Louis, then hold the other ruler at a 90-degree angle to the first, with one end at the angle of Louis and the other in the jugular area of the neck (Figure 8.2).

Assessment Techniques/ Normal Findings	Special Considerations

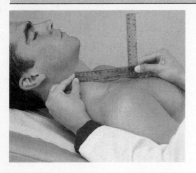

Figure 8.2 Assessment of central venous pressure.

• Observe neck for distention in jugular veins and raise horizontal ruler to top of height of distention. Read height from vertical ruler. Compare to normal distention of 3 cm above sternal angle when client is lying at a 45-degree angle.

Distention of neck veins is often seen with congestive heart failure, fluid overload, or pressure on superior vena cava.

8. Inspect carotid arteries.
Locate arteries in groove medial to sternocleidomastoid and lateral to trachea. With client lying at a 45-degree angle, check for pulsations. Confirm bilaterally visible pulsations. Help client return to upright position.

Bounding pulses may indicate fever, while the absence of a pulsation may indicate an obstruction internal or external to the artery.

9. Inspect hands and fingers.
• With client in sitting position, check hands and fingers. Confirm that fingertips are rounded and even and that fingernails are relatively flat and pink, with white crescents at the nail base.

Bilaterally clubbed fingertips and nails are characteristic of congenital heart disease, as well as cyanosis or infective endocarditis. Thin red lines in nailbeds are also associated with infective endocarditis. Fingertips and nails stained yellow could indicate a smoking habit, a primary contributor to atherosclerosis.

Assessment Techniques/ Normal Findings	Special Considerations

10. Inspect chest.

- Confirm even, regular, and unlabored respiratory pattern, without retractions.

Respiratory distress could be indicative of many disorders, including pulmonary edema, a severe complication of cardiovascular disease.

- Confirm veins in chest are evenly distributed and relatively flat.

Dilated, distended veins in chest indicate obstructive process such as obstruction of superior vena cava.

- Assess chest for bulges and masses. Confirm that intercostal spaces (ICS) and clavicles are even.

Bulges could indicate obstructions or aneurysms, while masses may indicate obstructions or tumors.

- Inspect entire chest for pulsations over the 5 key landmarks, first with client upright, then at 30-degree angle (Figure 8.3):

If entire precordium pulsates and shakes with each heartbeat, extreme valvular regurgitation or shunting may be present.

   Right sternal border (RSB), 2nd ICS

   Left sternal border (LSB), 2nd ICS

Pulsations could indicate pulmonary artery dilation or excessive blood flow.

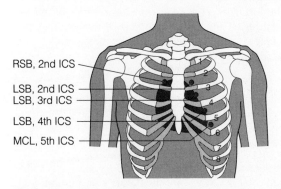

RSB, 2nd ICS
LSB, 2nd ICS
LSB, 3rd ICS
LSB, 4th ICS
MCL, 5th ICS

Figure 8.3   Five key landmarks in precordial cardiac assessment.

Assessment Techniques/ Normal Findings	Special Considerations
LSB, 3rd to 5th ICS	Pulsations may indicate right ventricular overload.
Midclavicular line (MCL), 5th ICS	
Epigastric area, below xiphoid process	
Confirm that point of maximal impulse (PMI) is located at MCL, 5th ICS	PMI is displaced laterally from MCL, 5th ICS, with left ventricular hypertrophy.
• Inspect entire chest for heaves or lifts over 5 key landmarks with client sitting upright and again at 30-degree angle.	Heave or lift found in LSB, 3rd to 5th ICS may indicate right ventricular hypertrophy or respiratory disease, such as pulmonary hypertension.

Alert!
Assess client's tolerance of different positions. Note especially shortness of breath and be prepared to alter your assessment sequence to meet the client's needs.

11. Inspect abdomen.
• Have client lie flat, if possible. Observe for pulsations over areas where major arteries are located, such as the aorta, the left and right renal arteries, and the right and left iliac arteries.
• Note pattern of fat distribution.

In lean clients, pulsations in epigastric area and peristaltic waves may be seen; these are normal. Readily visible prominent pulsations outside gastric area may be potentially life threatening.

Referral
Abnormal pulsations usually originate from aortic aneurysms and require immediate physician referral.

12. Inspect legs.
• Help client to a sitting position. Inspect legs for skin color. Verify that color is even and uniform.

Patches of lighter color may indicate circulatory compromise. Mottling indicates severe hemodynamic compromise.

Assessment Techniques/ Normal Findings	Special Considerations
• Assess hair distribution. Confirm that distribution is even without bare patches.	Patchy hair distribution is often a sign of circulatory compromise that has occurred over time. Ask client if hair distribution on legs has changed over time.

13. Inspect skeletal structure.

• Ask client to stand. Confirm that skeletal structure is free of deformities.	Scoliosis is associated with prolapsed mitral valve.
• Observe neck and extremities. Confirm proper proportions to torso.	Evaluate a tall, thin client with elongated neck and extremities for Marfan's syndrome.

Palpation

Palpate in each of the 5 key landmark areas with the client breathing normally, then breathing out, and holding breath, if possible. Start by palpating with the client sitting upright, then in the lowest position that the client can comfortably tolerate.

1. Place palm of right hand over RSB, 2nd ICS.
No pulsations, heaves, or vibratory sensations should be felt.

Pulsations or heaves in this area indicate presence of ascending aortic enlargement or aneurysm, aortic stenosis, or systemic hypertension.

2. Place hand on LSB, 2nd ICS.
No pulsations, heaves, or vibratory sensations should be felt except in very thin clients who are nervous.

Pulsations or heaves in this area are associated with pulmonary hypertension, pulmonary stenosis, right ventricular enlargement, atrial septal defect, enlarged left atrium, and large posterior left ventricular aneurysm.

Assessment Techniques/ Normal Findings	Special Considerations
3. Move hand to LSB, 3rd to 5th ICS. No pulsations, heaves, or vibratory sensations should be felt.	Pulsations or heaves in this area may indicate right ventricular enlargement or pressure overload, pulmonary stenosis, or pulmonary hypertension.
4. Place right hand over apex (MCL, 5th ICS). Confirm soft vibration or tapping sensation with each heartbeat, isolated to area of 1 cm diameter or less.	A heave indicates potential presence of increased right ventricular stroke volume or pressure and mild to moderate aortic regurgitation. A vibration palpated downward and lateral from normal PMI and/or greater than 1 cm could indicate left ventricular hypertrophy, severe left ventricular volume overload, or severe aortic regurgitation.
5. Palpate epigastric area, below xiphoid process.	Heaves or thrills suggest presence of elevated right ventricular volume and/or pressure overload.

6. Repeat palpation from Steps 1 to 5 with client at a 30-degree angle or supine.

Alert!

Place patients unable to lie flat at lowest angle tolerable. Stop assessment if physical distress is noted.

Confirm either no pulsation or faint taps in a localized area, and no thrills, heaves, or lifts in any of the 5 locations.

7. Palpate carotid pulses.

Alert!

Never palpate both carotid pulses simultaneously.

Assessment Techniques/ Normal Findings	Special Considerations
With client supine or sitting, ask client to look straight ahead and keep neck straight. Palpate each carotid pulse separately, ascertaining equal intensity, regular pattern, and strong, but not bounding, intensity.	Diminished or absent pulses could indicate carotid disease, dissecting ascending aneurysm, or (if both pulses are absent) asystole. For client in critical care with arterial line, obtain printout of arterial waveform.

8. Palpate for hepatojugular reflex.

- Position client in supine or low Fowler's position.
- Observe level of jugular vein pulsation. With your right hand flat, press slowly on the client's abdomen below the right costal margin.

Alert!
Do not press into abdomen with a sharp or rapid motion.

- Press for 30 to 60 seconds, while looking for sustained distention of jugular vein, then release. Confirm that distention diminishes quickly.	Distention is sustained with right-sided heart failure.

Auscultation

The position of the client affects data collected during auscultation. A full exam includes auscultation with the client sitting upright, leaning forward when upright, supine, and in the left lateral position.

Have client breathe normally. If you recognize abnormal sounds, have client slow respiration and note effect of inspiration and expiration on heart sounds; if desired, have client perform forced expiration.

Assessment Techniques/ Normal Findings	Special Considerations

Alert!

Assess client's ability to tolerate position changes and respiratory efforts. Stop if discomfort or distress is expressed or exhibited by client.

1. Auscultate chest with diaphragm of stethoscope.
Inch the stethoscope slowly across the chest and listen over each of the five key landmarks (Figure 8.4):

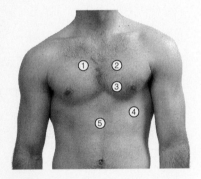

Figure 8.4 Five key landmarks for auscultation.

- At RSB, 2nd ICS, S_2 should be louder than S_1.
- At LSB, 2nd ICS, S_2 should be louder than S_1.
- At LSB, 3rd ICS, S_1 and S_2 should be relatively equal in intensity.
- At LSB, 4th ICS, S_1 should be louder than S_2.
- At apex (MCL, 5th ICS), S_1 should be louder than S_2.

Assessment Techniques/ Normal Findings	Special Considerations
2. Auscultate chest with bell of stethoscope. Place bell of stethoscope lightly on each of the five key landmarks. Start with S_3S_4 and listen for murmurs.	Low-pitched sounds are best auscultated with the bell.
3. Auscultate carotid arteries. • Use Doppler if pulse cannot be auscultated with stethoscope. • Ask client to breathe normally. You should hear movement of air and tracheal breath sounds, but not turbulent sounds like murmurs. • Ask client to briefly hold breath. Presence of heart tones is normal.	A bruit is most often associated with a narrowing or stricture of the artery, usually associated with atherosclerotic plaque.
4. Compare apical pulse to carotid pulse. Auscultate apical pulse while simultaneously palpating carotid pulse. The two pulses should be synchronous.	An apical pulse greater than the carotid rate indicates a pulse deficit. The rate, rhythm, and regularity must be evaluated.
5. Repeat auscultation with client leaning forward, supine, and in left lateral position.	

Strategy for Differentiating and Interpreting Heart Sounds

Sequence to Use During Auscultation

Remember to take your time when auscultating. Listen at all five sites and don't rush. You will need absolute quiet. If you hear more than S_1S_2, determine which sounds are S_1S_2 and then analyze the rest. Always follow the same auscultation strategy. The following is one possible sequence:

1. Use diaphragm of stethoscope to listen for S_1S_2 sounds, then listen for split S_1 and split S_2 sounds.

2. Use bell of stethoscope to assess for and to differentiate the S_3 and S_4 sounds from the split sounds. Listen also for the presence of summation gallop. Apply light rather than firm pressure on each landmark when using the bell to hear softer sounds.

3. Return to using the diaphragm to assess for murmurs from regurgitant valves, clicks, ejection sounds, snaps, and pericardial friction rubs.

4. Finish by using the bell to assess for murmurs of stenotic valves.

Interpreting Heart Sounds

Heart Sound	Cardiac Cycle Timing	Auscultation Site	Pitch	Effect of Respirations
S_1	Start of systole	Best at apex with diaphragm	High	Less intense with inspiratory effort
S_2	End of systole	Best at base of the heart in the aortic and pulmonic areas	High	Physiologic split may occur with inspiratory effort
Split S_1	Beginning of systole	If normal, at 2nd ICS, LSB; abnormal if heard at apex	High	Louder with inspiration
Split S_2	End of systole	Both at 2nd ICS; pulmonary component best at LSB, aortic at RSB with diaphragm	High	Louder on inspiration; paradoxical split only heard on inspiration
S_3	Early diastole right after S_2	Apex with bell; client in left lateral position, if possible	Low	Louder with inspiratory effort
S_4	Late diastole right before S_1	Apex with bell; client in left lateral position, if possible	Low	Louder with inspiratory effort
Clicks	Early systole	2nd ICS, RSB for aortic click and apex with diaphragm	High	Pulmonic click is softer with inspiratory effort
		2nd ICS, LSB for pulmonic click with diaphragm		
Snaps	Early diastole	3rd to 4th ICS, LSB with diaphragm	High	No effect
Rubs	Can occur at any time	Location varies; best heard with diaphragm	High, harsh, grating	Louder when breath is held

- A split S_1 sound consists of two sounds of equal intensity and very close together in sequence at the beginning of systole. (If an S_4 is present, the sounds are not of equal intensity.) There is only a brief pause between sounds, unlike the pause between S_1 and S_2. If you hear a split S_1 sound, answer the following questions:
  1. How wide is the split?
  2. Is it fixed, or does the respiratory cycle affect the wideness of the split?
  3. Are the split S_1 sounds of equal intensity or is one softer?
- A split S_2 sound is the same as a split S_1 sound, but occurs at the time you expect to hear the S_3 sound.
- A summation gallop is composed of $S_1S_2S_3S_4$ and sounds like a horse gallop. It is often associated with severe congestive heart failure.
- A pericardial friction rub can be very elusive and easily confused with murmurs. It may be found anywhere over the chest and precordium, and can be continuous or sporadic.

Nursing Diagnoses Commonly Associated with the Cardiovascular System

- **Cardiac output, decreased**—a state in which the blood pumped by an individual's heart is sufficiently reduced that it is inadequate to meet the needs of the body's tissues
- **Denial, ineffective**—a conscious or unconscious attempt to disavow the knowledge or meaning of an event to reduce anxiety/fear, to the detriment of health
- **Fluid volume, excess**—can be a significant outcome of cardiovascular ischemia or injury caused by myocardial infarction, or a sequela of chronic conditions such as heart failure or hepatic and renal disease
- **Gas exchange, impaired**—a state in which the individual experiences a decreased passage of oxygen and/or carbon dioxide between the alveoli of the lungs and the vascular septum
- **Pain, acute**—a state in which the individual reports discomfort or an uncomfortable sensation. This discomfort is whatever the person experiencing it says it is, and exists whenever he or she says it does.
- **Altered tissue perfusion, cardiovascular**—inability to provide adequate oxygen and nutrients to the myocardial tissue

Common Cardiovascular System Alterations

Congenital heart disease, electrical rhythm disturbances, myocardial infarction, myocardial ischemia, septal defects, valvular heart disease, ventricular hypertrophy.

Cardiovascular System Client Education

Help client promote cardiovascular health before the development of cardiovascular disease, and optimize and maintain the present level of cardiovascular health if cardiovascular disease is present. Discuss unmodifiable and modifiable risk factors and strategies for implementing permanent lifestyle changes.

Modifiable Risk Factors

Diet

To help client reduce or eliminate saturated fat from diet:

- Provide information that defines saturated fat, discusses its detrimental effects and lists foods containing saturated fats.
- Provide information on determining the fat content of processed foods.

To help client reduce or eliminate salt and MSG from diet:

- Provide information that describes the effect of salt and MSG and that lists foods that contain one or both.
- Provide information on salt alternatives and their correct use.

To help client understand need for fiber:

- Provide information that defines dietary fiber, its beneficial effects, and foods high in dietary fiber.

Inactive Lifestyle

- Help client define a well-balanced exercise program that includes aerobic activity designed to stimulate the heart without causing injury.
- Underscore need for supervision in developing an exercise program, to avoid injury and promote compliance.
- Help client see the value of regular exercise.

Elevated Body Fat Percentage

- Have lab work done to assess electrolytes, kidney function, total cholesterol, LDL, HDL, triglycerides, and uric acid before beginning an exercise and diet program. Undergo 12-lead ECG. Repeat tests throughout the program.
- Assess progress with body composition analysis every 2 months.
- Avoid crash or fad diets.

- Do not lose more than 1/2 pound of fat per week.
- Base success on body composition testing, reduction in inches, muscle tone, and increased energy and endurance, not weight loss.

Smoking

- Encourage smoker to quit; encourage nonsmoker not to begin.
- Help client understand that all types of smoking are harmful.
- Ensure that use of nicotine patches is supervised.

Stress

- Examine causes of stress.
- Provide information on stress reduction techniques and explore which is most beneficial and easily incorporated into the client's lifestyle.

Type A Behavior

- Discuss the characteristics of Type A behavior.
- Identify Type A behaviors the client might exhibit.
- Determine behaviors client feels able to modify.

Considerations for the Healthy Client

- Advise clients to inform dentists of the presence of murmurs and other cardiovascular problems.
- Discuss signs of a heart attack and when and how to activate emergency medical services (call 911).
- Instruct client to seek medical attention for the following signs of cardiovascular disorder: sudden weight gain or loss, palpitations, difficulty breathing with or without effort, peripheral swelling, new chronic headache, ringing in the ears.

Considerations for the Client with Cardiovascular Disease

- Review classic and atypical signs of cardiovascular disease.
- Review use of nitroglycerin, including dosage and need to inform physician if typical dosage does not relieve symptoms.
- Review signs of digitalis toxicity: nausea, blurring and other vision changes, loss of appetite, mentation changes. Advise client to inform physician if symptoms appear.
- Instruct clients on diuretics to increase intake of potassium-rich foods and take prescribed potassium replacements.
- Provide sources of information on sexual relations following a diagnosis of cardiovascular disease.

Cardiovascular System Physical Assessment Summary

Inspection

1. Position client.
2. Inspect face.
3. Inspect eyes.
4. Inspect lips.
5. Inspect earlobes.
6. Inspect head.
7. Inspect jugular veins.
8. Inspect carotid arteries.
9. Inspect hands and fingers.
10. Inspect chest.
11. Inspect abdomen.
12. Inspect legs.
13. Inspect skeletal structure.

Palpation

1. Place palm of right hand over RSB, 2nd ICS.
2. Place hand on LSB, 2nd ICS.
3. Move hand to LSB, 3rd to 5th ICS.
4. Place right hand over apex (MCL, 5th ICS).
5. Palpate epigastric area, below xiphoid process.
6. Repeat palpation from Steps 1 to 5 with client at a 30-degree angle or supine.
7. Palpate carotid pulses.
8. Palpate for hepatojugular reflex.

Auscultation

1. Auscultate chest with diaphragm of stethoscope.
2. Auscultate chest with bell of stethoscope.
3. Auscultate carotid arteries.
4. Compare apical pulse to carotid pulse.
5. Repeat auscultation with client leaning forward, supine, and in left lateral position.

Chapter 9

Assessing the Breasts and Axillae

Focused Interview

During the focused interview, you will be gathering information about the health of the breasts, how the client perceives her breasts, and how this affects her body image.

The physical examination of the breasts may be incorporated into the total body assessment along with the heart and lung assessment when the client is sitting and again when supine. Although much of this chapter's material assumes a female client, be sure to incorporate physical assessment of male breasts, perhaps during assessment of the thorax.

General Survey of Breasts and Axillae

1. Describe your breasts. How do they differ, if at all, from 3 months ago? 3 years ago?
2. Are you still menstruating? If so, describe any breast changes related to your normal menstrual cycle, such as tenderness, swelling, pain, or enlarged nodes. When was your last period?
3. Describe any changes in breast characteristics such as size, symmetry, shape, thickening, lumps, swelling, temperature, color of skin or vessels, or sensations (eg, tingling or tenderness). How long you have had them?
4. What medications are you taking?
5. How do you feel about your breasts?

Personal History

1. Have you ever had breast cancer, fibrocystic breast disease, or fibroadenoma?
2. Have you ever had breast surgery? If so, what and when? How has it affected you? Has it affected your sex life?

3. How old were you when you began menstruating?
4. Do you have children? How old were you when they were born?
5. Have you gone through menopause? If so, at what age? Were there any residual problems? Have you received hormone therapy during or since menopause?
6. Have you ever had a mammogram? When was your most recent one?
7. Have you had cancer in the endometrium, ovaries, colon or other body region?
8. Do you see your doctor on a regular basis for a physical exam?

Family History

1. Has your mother or a sister had breast cancer?
2. Has one of your grandmothers or an aunt had breast cancer?

Breast Self-Examination

1. Do you perform breast self-examination? If so, how often and at what time in your menstrual cycle?

Physical Assessment

- Gather the following equipment:

  centimeter ruler   gown

  gloves   small pillow or folded towel
- Follow universal precautions and wear gloves if any drainage is observed.
- Remember to use a friendly, yet matter-of-fact approach to help overcome any possible embarrassment on the part of the client.

Assessment Techniques/ Normal Findings	Special Considerations

Inspection

1. Position client.
Instruct client to sit comfortably and erect with arms at side and with gown around waist so both breasts are exposed.

Assessment Techniques/ Normal Findings	Special Considerations
2. Inspect and compare breast size and symmetry bilaterally. One breast may be slightly larger.	Obvious masses, flattening of breast in one area, skin dimpling, or recent size increase of one breast may indicate abnormal growth or inflammation.
3. Inspect skin color. Note any thickening, tautness, redness, rash, or ulceration.	Red, warm skin suggests inflammation. Peau d'orange skin indicates advanced cancer.
4. Inspect venous patterns. Confirm that venous patterns are similar bilaterally (more visible in pregnant or obese breast).	Pronounced unilateral venous patterns may indicate increased blood flow to a malignancy.
5. Inspect nipples for size, shape, color, direction, surface characteristics, and discharge. **Alert!** If any drainage is observed, use universal precautions and wear gloves. Confirm that nipples are almost equal in size and shape and of the same color as the areolae. They should be everted, flat, or inverted; pointing in the same direction (outward, slightly upward); and free of cracks, crust, erosions, ulcerations, pigment changes, or discharge.	Recent nipple retraction, inversion, or change in direction suggests malignancy. Further investigate bloody discharge, especially when accompanied by a mass (save discharge for cytological examination). Red, scaly, eczema-like area over nipple (possibly exuding fluid, scale, or crust) could indicate Paget's disease, especially if it persists more than a few weeks. Peau d'orange skin (often visible first on areola) suggests cancer. Breast-feeding may cause redness and/or fissures.
6. Observe breasts for bilateral pull on suspensory ligaments.	

Assessment Techniques/ Normal Findings	Special Considerations

Ask client to assume the following positions while you inspect breasts:

- Arms extended above head
- Hands pressed against hips
- Hands pushed together at waist level
- Leaning forward from waist

Assess whether breasts fall freely and evenly from chest.

Suspect breast cancer if breasts do not fall freely and evenly.

Palpation

1. Position client.

Ask client to lie supine. Cover breast not being palpated. Place small pillow or folded towel under side to be palpated, and position client's arm over her head.

2. Palpate skin texture of breasts. Confirm that skin texture is smooth and contour uninterrupted.

Thickened skin suggests an underlying carcinoma.

3. Palpate breasts.

- Using pads of first three fingers and a slightly rotary motion, press breast tissue against chest wall. Start at the periphery of the breast and palpate in large circles, proceeding to smaller circles until you reach the nipple. Be sure to palpate the entire breast, including the axillary tail.

The incidence of breast cancer is highest in the upper outer quadrant, including the axillary tail. Masses in the axillary tail must be distinguished from enlarged axillary lymph nodes.

Assessment Techniques/ Normal Findings	Special Considerations

- Palpate lightly at first, then deeper, with a firm, gentle touch, using a set pattern, as exemplified by the concentric circle pattern shown in Figure 9.1.

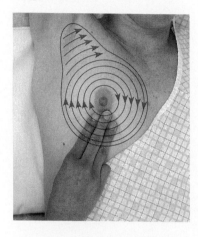

Figure 9.1   Palpating the breast.

- With pendulous breasts, place one hand under breast while pushing against breast tissue in downward motion with other hand, as shown in Figure 9.2.

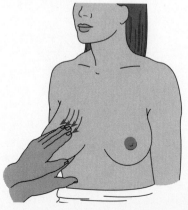

Figure 9.2   Palpating a pendulous breast.

Assessment Techniques/ Normal Findings	Special Considerations
• Confirm granular feel to breast tissue, with firm transverse ridge along lower edge of breast. Normal variations include the lobular feel of glandular tissue, and a fine granular feel in breast tissue of older women.	**Referral** Any hard, irregular, poorly circumscribed nodule fixed to skin or to underlying tissues suggests cancer and must be investigated further.
• Note where the woman is in her menstrual cycle so you can properly interpret changes such as breast tenderness.	
• If a mass is detected, document all of the following information:	
Location—describe using clock face method; state distance from nipple	
Size—state in centimeters	
Shape—describe as round, oval, regular, or irregular	
Consistency—state if soft, firm, or hard	
Tenderness—describe degree	
Mobility—Does the lump move, or is it fixed to skin or underlying tissue?	
Borders—Are the borders discrete or poorly defined?	
Presence or absence of dimpling or retraction	
Are any adjacent lymph nodes palpable?	

Assessment Techniques/ Normal Findings	Special Considerations

4. Palpate nipples and areolae.
- Compress tissue between your thumb and forefinger. Confirm that nipple is free of discharge and nontender, and that areola is free of masses.

Galactorrhea suggests endocrine disorders or medications, including tricyclic antidepressants, antihypertensive drugs, and estrogen. Unilateral discharge from one nipple or duct suggests a local lesion, possibly related to fibrocystic breast disease, an intraductal papilloma, or cancer.

5. Inspect and palpate axillae.
- Ask client to sit. Direct her to flex arm at elbow while you support it on your arm, as shown in Figure 9.3.

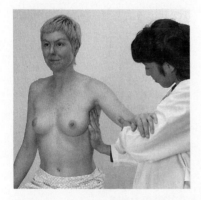

Figure 9.3　Palpating the axilla.

- Using palmar surface of your fingers, reach deep into axilla and gently palpate tissue against chest wall and underlying muscles of axilla, covering anterior border of axilla, central or medial aspect along rib cage, posterior border, and inner aspect of upper arm.

Enlarged, tender axillary lymph nodes indicate possible infection of breast, arm, or hand, or disease process. Hard, fixed nodes may suggest metastatic cancer or lymphoma.

Assessment Techniques/ Normal Findings	Special Considerations
• Confirm that axilla is free of redness, lumps, and rashes.	
• For clients who have had a wide local excision and/or mastectomy, use same technique to palpate remaining tissue on chest wall. Do not assume that tissue is disease-free.	Note that removal of a lump or breast does not ensure that remaining tissue is free of disease.

Examination of Male Breast

1. Inspect breasts. Confirm that breasts are flat and free of lumps and rashes.	Breast cancer in males is rare, but it does occur, and incidence increases after age 65.
2. Palpate breasts. • Ask client to lie supine. Confirm that breast feels like thin disc of tissue under a flat nipple and areola. • Compress nipple between fingers. Confirm absence of discharge.	Gynecomastia occurs temporarily in some adolescents, as well as with some hormonal medications and diseases. Breast cancer in males is identified as a hard, irregular nodule often fixed to the nipple and underlying tissue. Nipple discharge may also be present.
• Palpate axilla for nodes in the same manner as in the female.	Swelling of the axillary lymph nodes suggests infection.

Common Breast and Axilla Alterations

Carcinoma of the breast, duct ectasia, fibroadenoma, fibrocystic breast disease, intraductal papilloma.

Nursing Diagnoses Commonly Associated with Breasts and Axillae

- **Body image disturbance**—viewing oneself differently as a result of actual or perceived changes in body structure or function
- **Dysfunctional grieving**—state in which an individual reacts to an actual, anticipated, or perceived loss of a significant person, ideal, status, object, or body part with an absent, delayed, exaggerated, or prolonged response
- **Ineffective breast feeding**

- **Ineffective individual coping**
- **Knowledge deficit related to lack of information about breast self-examination**
- **Anxiety related to the diagnosis of cancer**
- **Pain related to metastasis**

Breast and Axilla Client Education

Discuss breast wellness and self-examination.

Promoting Healthy Breasts

All women should know they are at risk for breast cancer and should be familiar with risk factors. Focus on modifiable risk factors and self-care practices. Clients need to be aware of screening and detection measures.

- Identify breast cancer risk factors summarized in Table 9.1.

Table 9.1   Summary of Risk Factors for Breast Cancer

Factor	Higher risk	Lower risk
Age	≥40	<40
History of cancer in one breast	Yes	No
Family history of premenopausal bilateral breast cancer	Yes	No
Country of residence	North America Northern Europe	Asia Africa
Any first-degree relative with breast cancer	Yes	No
History of fibrocystic condition with atypical hyperplasia	Yes	No
Alcohol consumption	>9 drinks/wk	<9 drinks/wk
History of primary cancer in ovary or endometrium	Yes	No
Radiation to chest	Large doses	Minimal exposure
Socioeconomic class	Upper	Lower
Age at first full-term pregnancy	>30	<20
Oophorectomy	Yes	No
Postmenopausal body build	Obese	Thin
Race	White	Black
Age at menarche	Early	Late
Age at menopause	Late	Early
U.S. place of residence	Urban northern	Rural southern

- Identify self-care practices that reduce cancer risk:

  Perform breast self-examination monthly after age 20

  Avoid obesity

  Reduce dietary fat

  Reduce alcohol intake

  Have oral contraceptive use monitored by a physician

  Have supplemental estrogen use monitored by a physician
- Have regular physical examinations every 3 years from age 20 to 40, then every year thereafter.
- Obtain a baseline mammography between 35 to 39 years of age. Have regular follow-up mammograms every 2 years if not at risk, and every year if at risk and age 50 or older.
- Wear a supportive bra when exercising.
- Report to a physician any changes in breasts or axillae that deviate from normal patterns, such as lumps, dimpling, deviation, recent nipple retraction, irregular shape, edema, or discharge.
- Use American Cancer Society resources for cancer information.

Breast Self-Examination

1. When the exam is complete, assess the client's knowledge of breast self-examination. Have the client tell you when she performs the exam, how often, and what she looks and palpates for. Then have her demonstrate her technique to you.
2. Teach client to observe breasts in front of a mirror, in good lighting, in four positions: arms relaxed at sides, arms lifted over head, hands pressed against hips, and hands pressed together at waist, leaning forward.

   Instruct client to look at each breast individually and then to compare them, observing for lumps, dimpling, deviation, recent nipple retraction, irregular shape, edema, discharge, asymmetry, or other abnormalities.
3. Teach client to palpate both breasts while standing or sitting, with one hand behind head. Show her how to use pads of fingers to palpate all areas of breast, using concentric circles. Instruct client to press breast tissue gently against chest wall and to palpate axillary tail.
4. Instruct client to repeat palpation lying down. Suggest she fold a towel under shoulder and back on side to be palpated and keep the hand under her head.
5. Teach client to palpate areolae and nipples. Show her how to compress nipple to check for discharge.

6. Remind client to use a calendar to keep a record of breast self-examination. Teach her to perform breast self-examination at the same time each month, usually five days after the onset of menses when hormonal influence on tissue is less.

Breast and Axilla Physical Assessment Summary

Inspection

1. Position client.
2. Inspect and compare breast size and symmetry bilaterally.
3. Inspect skin color.
4. Inspect venous patterns.
5. Inspect nipples for size, shape, color, direction, surface characteristics, and discharge.
6. Observe breasts for bilateral pull on suspensory ligaments.

Palpation

1. Position client.
2. Palpate skin texture of breasts.
3. Palpate breasts.
4. Palpate nipples and areolae.
5. Inspect and palpate axillae.

Examination of Male Breast

1. Inspect breasts.
2. Palpate breasts.

Chapter 10

Assessing the Abdomen

Focused Interview

Question the client about patterns, problems, and lifestyle and environmental conditions that might affect the abdomen. You will want to assess the client's developmental stage, self-care practices, cultural and environmental variations, and the psychosocial implications of food during the focused interview.

1. Describe your appetite. Has your appetite changed in the last 24 hours, month, year? Has your weight changed? What have you eaten in the last 24 hours, including snacks, and how much of each item? Is this typical?

2. How much coffee, tea, cola, alcohol, and chocolate do you consume daily?

3. Do you experience nausea or vomiting? If so, how frequently, and when was the last occurrence? What was the cause? What do you do to relieve the symptoms? When you vomit, what comes up and how much?

4. Do you have difficulty chewing or swallowing food? Do you wear dentures? Do you have any crowns? Do your gums bleed easily?

5. Describe your bowel habits, noting frequency. What is the color and consistency of your stool? Do you experience pain, notice blood, have diarrhea, or experience constipation? If so, what is the cause and what do you do to correct it?

6. Do you work with chemical irritants?

7. Have you traveled recently? Where?

8. Describe your stress level. Are you coping well?

9. Do you have abdominal pain now? Where? Is it constant? Does it radiate? What do you think is the cause? How do you relieve it?

Physical Assessment

- Gather the following equipment:

drape	ruler
examination gown	skin-marking pen
examination light	stethoscope
gloves	tape measure

- Before beginning assessment, ask client to void.
- Have client lie supine with small pillows under head and knees. Drape gowns over chest, pelvic area, and legs, with abdomen exposed. Client remains in this position unless otherwise indicated. Stand on right side of client unless otherwise indicated.
- Determine if abdominal pain is present before proceeding, and examine the painful area last.
- Use universal precautions and put on gloves if you notice open skin areas.

Assessment Techniques/ Normal Findings	Special Considerations

Inspection

1. Determine contour of abdomen.
Observe profile of abdomen between costal margins and symphysis pubis. Confirm flat, rounded, or scaphoid abdomen.

Protuberant abdomen—normal in pregnancy—may indicate obesity or ascites in a nonpregnant client.

2. Observe location of umbilicus. Confirm that umbilicus is in center of abdomen, is inverted or protruding, and is clean and free of drainage or inflammation.

Protruding or displaced umbilicus—normal in pregnancy—may indicate abdominal mass or distended urinary bladder in a nonpregnant adult. Accompanying drainage or inflammation could indicate infectious process.

Referral

A client with drainage from the umbilicus following laparoscopic surgery should be referred to the physician immediately.

Assessment Techniques/ Normal Findings	Special Considerations

3. Observe skin of abdomen.

- Confirm that color and luster of skin is consistent with rest of body.

Taut and glistening skin may indicate abdominal ascites. *Striae* are common in obesity, pregnancy, and ascites.

- Observe location and characteristics of scars.

Scars indicate surgery and possibility of underlying adhesions.

4. Observe abdomen for symmetry, bulging, or masses.

- First observe abdomen while standing at client's side; then observe while standing at foot of bed or table, comparing sides. Return to client's side and shine light across abdomen. Observe abdomen from sitting or kneeling position. Check for symmetry and bulging or masses.

Light produces a shadow on small bulges or masses.

A bulge could indicate a tumor, cyst, or hernia.

- Ask client to take a deep breath and raise head off pillow, then repeat inspection.

Deep breathing and head-raising accentuate masses.

5. Observe abdominal wall for movement.

In a thin adult, pulsations of the abdominal aorta below the xiphoid process are common. Peristaltic waves are normal with a well-relaxed muscle wall.

Marked pulsations could indicate aortic aneurysm or increased pulse pressure. Increased peristaltic activity could indicate gastroenteritis or obstructive process.

Auscultation

Alert!

Auscultate before percussing or palpating to avoid altering peristaltic action.

Assessment Techniques/ Normal Findings	Special Considerations

1. Auscultate for bowel sounds.
Using diaphragm of stethoscope, begin in right lower quadrant (RLQ) over ileocecal junction of intestines and move through all quadrants (Figure 10.1). Count sounds for at least 60 seconds, noting both character and frequency. Normal sounds are irregular, gurgling, and high-pitched, occurring 5 to 30 times per minute. *Borborygmi* occurs in clients who have not eaten in a few hours.

Alert!
Always auscultate all quadrants for at least 5 minutes total before documenting absent bowel sounds.

Hyperactive sounds—loud, high-pitched, and rushing—are common with gastroenteritis and diarrhea. Hypoactive sounds often follow abdominal surgery or end-stage obstruction. Absent sounds may indicate a paralytic ileus.

Referral
Clients with intestinal obstruction or paralytic ileus require immediate medical attention.

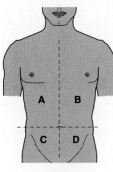

A
Right Upper Quadrant
Liver and gallbladder
Pyloric sphincter
Duodenum
Head of pancreas
Right adrenal gland
Portion of right kidney
Hepatic flexure of colon
Portions of ascending
    and transverse colon

B
Left Upper Quadrant
Left lobe of liver
Spleen
Stomach
Body of pancreas
Left adrenal gland
Portion of left kidney
Splenic flexure of colon
Portions of transverse
    and descending colon

C
Right Lower Quadrant
Lower pole of right kidney
Cecum and appendix
Portion of ascending
    colon
Ovary and uterine tube
Right spermatic cord
Right ureter

D
Left Lower Quadrant
Lower pole of left kidney
Sigmoid colon
Portion of descending
    colon
Ovary and uterine tube
Left spermatic cord
Left ureter

Midline
Aorta
Bladder
Uterus

O = Umbilicus

Figure 10.1   Organs of the four abdominal quadrants.

Assessment Techniques/ Normal Findings	Special Considerations
2. Auscultate for vascular sounds. Using stethoscope bell, listen over abdominal aorta, renal, iliac, and femoral arteries (Figure 10.2). Auscultatory sounds of the abdomen are listed in Table 10.1.	Bruits heard during systole and diastole may indicate partial arterial occlusion. A venous hum usually indicates increased portal tension. A friction rub usually indicates tumor, infection, infarct, or peritonitis, and requires further medical evaluation.

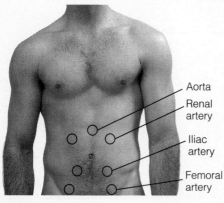

Aorta
Renal artery
Iliac artery
Femoral artery

Figure 10.2 Auscultatory areas for vascular sounds.

TABLE 10.1 Abdominal Sounds Heard upon Auscultation

Abdominal Sound	Characteristics
Bowel sounds	Movement of the gastrointestinal tract produces irregular, gurgling, high-pitched sounds.
Borborygmi	Similar to bowel sounds, but more frequent. Borborygmi signals increased movement of the gastrointestinal tract and produces loud, high-pitched, gurgling sounds. Commonly heard with hunger and diarrhea.
Venous hum	A soft, low-pitched, vibrating sound. This bruit-like sound is an indication of liver or splenic disease.
Bruit	A blowing or swishing sound indicating an obstruction in the vessel.
Friction rub	A rough, grating sound indicating irritation of the peritoneum.

Assessment Techniques/ Normal Findings	Special Considerations

Percussion

1. Percuss the 4 quadrants of the abdomen to determine amount of tympany and dullness.
Percuss in orderly pattern, as shown in Figure 10.3. Confirm tympany over underlying structures holding air, dullness over liver and spleen. Table 10.2 lists percussion sounds of the abdomen.

Dullness may indicate enlarged uterus, distended urinary bladder, or ascites.

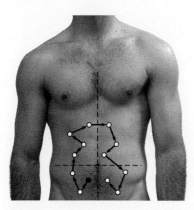

Figure 10.3   Percussion pattern for abdomen.

TABLE 10.2   Abdominal Sounds Heard upon Percussion

Abdominal Sound	Characteristics
Tympany	A loud, hollow sound should be obtained in the four quadrants. They are loudest over the gastric bubble and intestines.
Dullness	A short, high-pitched sound heard over liver, spleen, and distended bladder.
Hyperresonance	Louder than tympany. Heard over air-filled or distended intestines.
Flat	A very soft, short, abrupt sound. This is heard when no air is present in the structure, as over muscle, bone, or tumor mass.

Assessment Techniques/ Normal Findings	Special Considerations

2. Percuss the liver.
Determine upper and lower borders of liver.

- Begin at level of umbilicus and percuss toward rib cage along extended right midclavicular line, (Figure 10.4). Tympany changes to dullness at lower liver border (usually costal margin). Mark with skin-marking pen.

Dullness below costal margin suggests liver enlargement or downward displacement from respiratory disease.

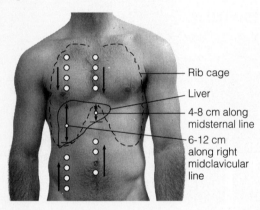

Rib cage

Liver

4-8 cm along midsternal line

6-12 cm along right midclavicular line

Figure 10.4 Percussion pattern for liver.

- Percuss downward from 4th intercostal space along right midclavicular line. Resonance changes to dullness at upper border of liver (usually at 6th intercostal space). Mark the point.
- Confirm distance of 5 to 10 cm between midclavicular marks.
- Repeat steps above along midsternal line. Confirm distance of 4 to 9 cm between midsternal marks.

Dullness above 5th or 6th intercostal space could indicate enlarged liver, upward displacement from ascites, or abdominal mass.

Assessment Techniques/ Normal Findings	Special Considerations
• Determine movement of liver with breathing: Ask client to take a deep breath and hold it. Percuss upward along extended right midclavicular line. Confirm that lower liver border descends about 1 inch.	Liver movement is diminished with an atelectasis or pneumothorax of right lung.
3. Percuss to determine size and location of spleen. Percuss left side of abdomen posterior to midaxillary line. Expect small area of splenic dullness from 6th to 10th intercostal space.	Splenic dullness at left anterior axillary line indicates *splenomegaly* and is perceptible before enlarged spleen is palpable.
4. Percuss gastric bubble. Percuss area between left costal margin and midsternal line extended below xiphoid process. Listen for low-pitched tympany to determine area of stomach.	A dull percussion sound suggests stomach mass. A very loud sound and an increased area suggest gastric dilation.

Palpation

Alert!
Identify painful areas before proceeding and palpate those areas last.

1. Lightly palpate abdomen. Place palmar surface of hand on abdomen with fingers extended and lightly press into abdomen with fingers. Move over all quadrants by lifting hand and placing it in another area. **Do not** drag or slide. Confirm soft, smooth, nontender, and pain-free abdomen.	Muscle tightness or guarding may indicate abdominal pain. Identify superficial masses. Note that abdominal pain from an organ is often referred to the surface of the abdomen or back.

Assessment Techniques/ Normal Findings	Special Considerations
2. Palpate abdomen using moderate pressure.	Masses, tumors, or intestinal obstructions may be palpated. A distended urinary bladder will be palpable above symphysis pubis as a smooth, tense mass.
• Following procedure in Step 1, palpate in all quadrants with pressure to depress abdomen about 2 inches.	
• Use bimanual technique for a large or obese abdomen.	In pregnant women, the uterus is palpable, with the height or placement of fundus influenced by week of gestation.
• Identify size of underlying organs and confirm absence of tenderness or masses. Note: The pancreas is nonpalpable.	A mass in the LLQ may be feces in colon. A vaguely palpable sensation of fullness in epigastric region may be pancreatic in origin.
3. Attempt to palpate liver. Standing on client's right side, place left hand under lower portion of rib cage at ribs 11 and 12. Ask client to relax into your left hand, and then lift the rib cage. Place your right hand gently but firmly into abdomen with an upward and inward thrust along costal margin, as shown in Figure 10.5. Ask client to take deep breath while you try to palpate lower edge of liver with right hand (usually only palpable in thin clients). If felt, confirm that liver is smooth, firm, and nontender, and that client has no pain.	Pain on palpation indicates gallbladder disease, acute hepatitis, or enlarged liver associated with congestive heart failure. A nodular liver indicates a metastatic carcinoma or cirrhosis. All of these conditions require further medical evaluation.

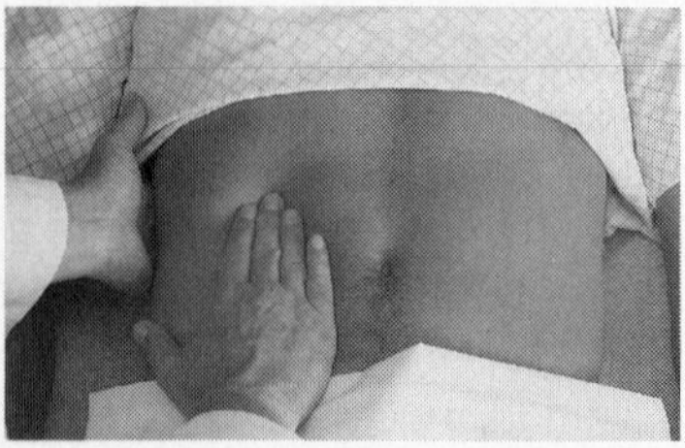

Figure 10.5 Palpating the liver.

Assessment Techniques/ Normal Findings	Special Considerations

4. Attempt to palpate spleen.
Standing on client's right side, place left hand beneath left lower rib cage and elevate cage, moving spleen anteriorly. Press fingertips of right hand into left costal margin area of client, as shown in Figure 10.6. Ask client to take a slow, deep breath through the mouth. As diaphragm descends, feel for spleen moving toward fingertips of right hand (usually not palpable).

Palpable spleen, which is usually greatly enlarged, is very sensitive and fragile. Splenomegaly occurs with acute infections, such as mononucleosis.

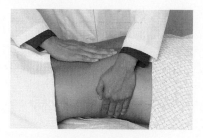

Figure 10.6   Palpating the spleen.

Additional Procedures

1. Palpate aorta for pulsations.

Alert!
Do not palpate a strong, wide abdominal pulsation.

Press fingertips firmly and deeply into upper abdomen to left of midline below xiphoid process. Confirm normal adult aortic width of 3 cm.

Obesity and abdominal masses will make aortic palpation difficult. A widened aorta may suggest an aneurysm.

Assessment Techniques/ Normal Findings	Special Considerations
2. Palpate for rebound tenderness. Hold hand at 90-degree angle to abdominal wall in an area of no pain or discomfort. Slowly and steadily, press fingers deeply into abdomen. Then rapidly remove fingers.	A sharp, stabbing pain as compressed structures return to precompressed state (a positive *Blumberg sign*) indicates peritoneal irritation. RLQ pain when pressure occurs in LLQ (a positive *Rovsing's sign*) may be due to peritoneal irritation or appendicitis. Refer to a physician immediately.
3. Percuss abdomen for ascites. • Percuss at midline and determine tympany sound, then percuss toward lateral aspects and listen for dullness. Mark skin, identifying possible levels of fluid. • Alternately, position client on right or left side and percuss abdomen. Confirm tympany at superior level and dullness at inferior level. • Measure abdominal girth with tape measure if ascites is suspected.	Ascites is common in clients with congestive heart failure, cirrhosis of the liver, or renal disease.

Nursing Diagnoses Commonly Associated with the Gastrointestinal System

- **Bowel incontinence**—state in which an individual experiences a change in normal bowel habits characterized by involuntary passage of stool
- **Constipation**—state in which an individual experiences a change in normal bowel habits characterized by a decrease in frequency and/or passage of hard, dry stools
- **Diarrhea**—state in which an individual experiences a change in normal bowel habits characterized by the frequent passage of loose, fluid, unformed stools

Common Gastrointestinal Tract Alterations

Nutritional Imbalances

Malnutrition, obesity, overweight.

Eating Disorders

Anorexia nervosa, bulimia nervosa.

Ulcers

Peptic ulcer, gastric ulcer, duodenal ulcer, ulcerative colitis.

Inflammatory Processes

Esophagitis, gastritis, enteritis, cholecystitis, peritonitis, hepatitis, pancreatitis, Chrohn's disease.

Abdominal Hernias

Umbilical hernia, ventral hernia, hiatal hernia.

Cancers

Esophageal cancer, stomach cancer, colorectal cancer.

Gastrointestinal System Client Education

Explain the importance of diet and preventive health care for abdominal wellness.

Diet

- Eat a balanced diet, including proteins, fats, carbohydrates, fresh fruit, and vegetables.
- Maintain regular bowel habits through proper diet and fiber consumption rather than with laxatives and enemas.
- Store and prepare food properly.
- Identify and decrease or eliminate foods that cause constipation, diarrhea, flatus, belching, or nausea, or that otherwise irritate the gastrointestinal system.

Preventive Health Care

- Know cancer warning signs specific to the gastrointestinal system:
  Change in bowel or bladder habits
  Unusual bleeding or discharge
  Indigestion or difficulty swallowing
- Avoid obesity.
- Control stress with healthy strategies, not smoking, food, drugs, and alcohol.
- Use medications correctly and know their side effects.

Abdomen Physical Assessment Summary

Inspection

1. Determine contour of abdomen.
2. Observe location of umbilicus.
3. Observe skin of abdomen.
4. Observe abdomen for symmetry, bulging, or masses.
5. Observe abdominal wall for movement.

Auscultation

1. Auscultate for bowel sounds.
2. Auscultate for vascular sounds.

Percussion

1. Percuss the 4 quadrants of abdomen to determine amount of tympany and dullness.
2. Percuss the liver.
3. Percuss to determine size and location of spleen.
4. Percuss gastric bubble.

Palpation

1. Lightly palpate abdomen.
2. Palpate abdomen using moderate pressure.
3. Attempt to palpate liver.
4. Attempt to palpate spleen.

Additional Procedures

1. Palpate aorta for pulsations.
2. Palpate for rebound tenderness.
3. Percuss abdomen for ascites.

Chapter 11

Assessing the Urinary System

Focused Interview

The examination of the urinary system is incorporated into other segments of the physical assessment because the organs of the urinary system are distributed among the retroperitoneal space, abdomen, and genitals. Be sure to start the interview by asking about the client's normal patterns before focusing on any deviations from normal.

General Health of the Urinary System

1. How frequently and how much do you normally urinate? Have you noticed any recent changes in frequency or volume?
2. Any recent changes in quality of urine, eg, cloudiness, odor, or color? Describe change and its predictability.
3. Is urine bloody? If so, have you fallen recently? Have you noticed any clots, stones, or other material in your urine?
4. Do you or any family member have a history of kidney disease or urinary problems? If so, when and how was it treated?
5. Do you have multiple sclerosis or Parkinson's disease? Have you suffered a spinal cord injury or stroke? If so, what, when, and how are you being treated?
6. Do you have cardiovascular disease? If so, what type, when was it diagnosed, and how are you being treated?
7. Are you currently taking any medication? Describe type, dose, and frequency. Why are you taking medication?
8. Describe your diet in a typical day, including how much you eat and drink. Do you take any dietary supplements?

9. Any pain or discomfort in back, sides, or abdomen? Please describe location, severity, timing, and predictability. What aggravates or alleviates the symptoms?

10. When was your last urine analysis and blood work evaluating kidney function? Do you know the results?

11. Do you have urinary problems that cause you embarrassment or anxiety? Have they affected social, personal, or sexual relationships?

Elimination Patterns

1. When you void, do you feel you are able to empty your bladder completely? If not, describe your feeling.

2. Are you always able to control urination? Have you ever urinated by accident?

3. Do you get up at night to urinate? Is there a predictable pattern?

4. Do you have difficulty starting to urinate? Does your urine flow continuously or does it start and stop? Do you need to strain or push to empty your bladder?

5. Do you ever have pain, burning, or other discomfort before, during, or after urination? If so, describe discomfort, location, timing, and predictability.

Physical Assessment

- Gather the following equipment:

  drape   gloves

  examination gown   specimen container

  examination light   stethoscope

- Before beginning physical assessment, have client empty the bladder and produce a urine specimen. Explain proper collection of specimen. Send specimen to the laboratory.

Assessment Techniques/ Normal Findings	Special Considerations

General Appearance

1. Position client.
Begin with client supine with abdomen exposed from nipple line to pubis.

Assessment Techniques/ Normal Findings	Special Considerations
2. Assess general appearance. • Confirm that client is alert, oriented, and not in distress. • Check skin for color, hydration, scales, masses, indentations, and scars.	Persons with kidney disorders frequently look tired and complain of fatigue. Other clues include pulmonary edema, peripheral edema, and pruritus. Elevated nitrogenous wastes in blood contribute to mental confusion.

Abdomen

1. Inspect abdomen color, contour, symmetry, and distention. • Inspect abdomen from side and foot of examination table using tangential light. Confirm that abdomen is not distended, is relatively symmetrical, and is free of bruises, masses, and swelling.	Abdominal distention could indicate polycystic kidney disease, acute pyelonephritis, hepatic disease, and displacement of abdominal organs.
• Observe breathing pattern.	Abdominal pressure can alter breathing.
• Inspect suprapubic area for distended bladder.	A distended bladder could indicate need and potential inability to void.

Kidneys and Flanks

1. Position client. Have client sit facing away from you with back exposed.	
2. Inspect color and symmetry of costovertebral angles and flanks. Confirm that color and symmetry are even.	A protrusion or elevation over a costovertebral angle occurs when a kidney is grossly enlarged or a mass is present. Carefully correlate this finding to other diagnostic cues as you proceed with the assessment.

Assessment Techniques/ Normal Findings	Special Considerations
3. Gently palpate areas over costovertebral angles. **Alert!** Do not palpate if client indicates pain or discomfort in pelvic region or if tumor is suspected. Palpate one side, then the other. Observe client's reaction. Ask client to describe any sensation. Confirm that client feels no discomfort. Assess temperature.	Pain, discomfort, or tenderness could indicate polycystic formation, pyelonephritis, or other disorders causing kidney enlargement. When questioned, the client will complain of a dull, steady ache. Sharp, sudden, intermittent pain could indicate a ruptured cyst in kidney. Chills, fever, nausea, and vomiting combined with tender, red, and warm costovertebral angle area could indicate an inflamed or infected kidney. Excruciating pain or dull, aching pain, sometimes radiating from flanks to lower abdomen, labium/scrotum, or upper thigh could indicate calculi in kidney or upper ureter. **Referral** Be alert for hydroureter if client is in severe pain and has hematuria or oliguria, along with nausea and vomiting. Seek medical collaboration immediately.
4. Use blunt or indirect percussion to further assess kidneys. **Alert!** Do not percuss if client indicates pain, discomfort, or tenderness. • Place left palm flat over left costovertebral angle and thump with ulnar surface of right fist. Ask client to describe sensation. Repeat on right side. • Confirm that client does not feel pain or tenderness.	Pain or discomfort during and after blunt percussion suggests kidney disease. Correlate with other assessment findings.

Assessment Techniques/ Normal Findings	Special Considerations

Left Kidney

1. Attempt to palpate lower pole of left kidney.

Alert!

Do not attempt deep kidney palpation or "capture" unless experienced or supervised by experienced practitioner. Deep kidney palpation should not be done on clients who have had a recent kidney transplant or an abdominal aortic aneurysm.

- Have client lie supine. Standing at client's right side, reach over client and place left hand between posterior rib cage and left flank. Place right hand on left upper quadrant of abdomen, lateral and parallel to left rectus muscle just below costal margin.

- Have client take a deep breath. As client inhales, lift flank with left hand and press deeply with right hand to attempt to palpate lower pole of kidney. Assess size, contour, consistency, and sensation (Figure 11.1).

Kidneys large enough to palpate could indicate neoplasms and polycystic disease. Otherwise, they are rarely palpable.

Note that an enlarged kidney feels smooth and rounded; an enlarged spleen feels sharper, with a more delineated edge.

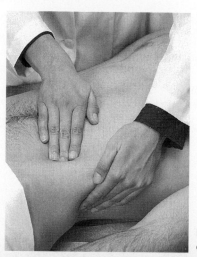

Figure 11.1 Palpating the lower pole of the left kidney.

Assessment Techniques/ Normal Findings	Special Considerations

2. Attempt to "capture" left kidney.

- Stand on client's right side with hands positioned as in Step 1. Have client take a deep breath and hold it. As client inhales, attempt to "capture" kidney between your hands.

- Have client slowly exhale, then briefly hold breath, while you release pressure of your fingers to let "captured" kidney move back into position. Confirm that kidney surface feels rounded, smooth, firm, and nontender.

Right Kidney

1. Attempt to palpate lower pole of right kidney.

- Standing on client's right side, place left hand under back parallel to right 12th rib, with fingertips reaching for costovertebral angle. Place right hand on right upper quadrant of abdomen, lateral to right rectus muscle, just below right costal margin.

- Have client take a deep breath. As client inhales, lift flank with left hand and press deeply with right hand to feel for lower pole of kidney.

2. Attempt to "capture" right kidney.
See Step 2 for left kidney.

Gross enlargement could indicate polycystic disease or carcinoma. Note that an enlarged kidney feels smooth and rounded; an enlarged liver is closer to midline and has a sharper border.

Nursing Diagnoses Commonly Associated with the Urinary System

- **Altered urinary elimination**—a disturbance in urine elimination
- **Urinary incontinence, functional**—inability to reach toilet in time because of environmental, psychosocial, or physical factors
- **Urinary incontinence, reflex**—urine involuntarily lost due to spinal cord damage
- **Urinary incontinence, stress**—urine loss of less than 50 ml occurring with increased abdominal pressure
- **Urinary incontinence, total**—related to urologic pathology
- **Urinary incontinence, urge**—significant volume fluids consumed in short period of time or bladder with diminished capacity
- **Urinary retention**—incomplete emptying of the bladder

Common Urinary System Alterations

Bladder cancer, glomerulonephritis, renal calculi, renal failure, renal tumor, urinary tract infection.

Urinary System Client Education

Discuss general care of the urinary system, bladder infection prevention, and cancer prevention for the urinary tract.

Promoting General Health

- Drink at least 8 glasses of water and other fluids daily. Moderate intake of alcohol, caffeinated or carbonated beverages.
- Moderate intake of foods containing baking powder and baking soda.
- Use over-the-counter drugs containing phenacetin in moderation.

Preventing Bladder Infections

- Drink plenty of water.
- Maintain proper pH of urine by consuming meat, eggs, cheese, whole grains, cranberries, prunes, and plums.
- Avoid bubble bath, scented tissue, perfumed soap, and other urethral irritants.
- Urinate immediately after sexual intercourse.
- *Females:* Clean perineum from front to back to avoid contamination of urethra. Wear cotton underwear. Avoid using diaphragms for contraception.

Preventing Urinary Tract Cancer

- Know urinary tract cancer risk factors: smoking, exposure to chemicals used in textile and rubber industries, and exposure to *Schistosoma haemotobium* parasite.
- Know renal cell carcinoma risk factors: males over 35 who smoke, use of analgesics containing phenacetin, and exposure to asbestos, cadmium, and gasoline.
- Seek immediate medical attention for abdominal mass or distended abdomen.
- Seek medical advice for 10- to 20-pound short-term weight loss, changes in urinary elimination patterns, or persistent lower back or flank pain.

Urinary System Physical Assessment Summary

General Appearance

Abdomen

1. Inspect abdomen color, contour, symmetry, and distention.

Kidneys and Flanks

1. Position client.
2. Inspect color and symmetry of costovertebral angles and flanks.
3. Gently palpate area over costovertebral angles.
4. Use blunt or indirect percussion to further assess kidneys.

Left Kidney

1. Attempt to palpate lower pole of left kidney.
2. Attempt to "capture" left kidney.

Right Kidney

1. Attempt to palpate lower pole of right kidney.
2. Attempt to "capture" right kidney.

Assessing the Reproductive System

Focused Interview

Ask the following questions to gather information about reproductive health and sexual functioning.

Male Clients

Reproductive Health

1. What concerns about your reproductive health do you have now or have you had in the past?
2. Have you noticed blisters, ulcers, sores, warts, rashes, swelling, redness, lumps, or masses on your penis, scrotum, or surrounding areas? Describe. When did you first notice this? What treatments have you tried?
3. Have you noticed any unusual discharge from your penis? Of what color? Is there any odor? Is it a small, moderate, or large amount? When did you first notice it? Is there burning or pain with the discharge?
4. Have you noticed any pain, tenderness, or soreness in the areas of your penis or scrotum? Describe it (eg, dull, radiating, continuous). What makes the pain better or worse?
5. Have you had unusual itching in your genital area? Where? Have you noticed any rashes, scaling, or lumps?
6. Have you had surgery on any reproductive organ? If so, what was the surgery?

Sexual Function

1. Are you able to be sexually aroused? Has this ability changed recently or over time?

2. Can you achieve and maintain an erection? Are you satisfied with the length of time it takes to achieve and maintain an erection?

3. Are you able to achieve orgasm? Are you satisfied with your ability to control the timing of your orgasms?

Female Clients

Reproductive Health

1. What concerns about your reproductive health do you have now or have you had in the past?

2. Have you noticed any rashes, blisters, ulcers, sores, or warts, swelling or redness on your genital area or surrounding areas?

3. Have you felt any lumps or masses in your genital area or surrounding area? If so, please describe its location, size, and whether it's soft or hard, movable, or painful. Have you noticed any change in it since it developed? What treatments have you tried?

4. Have you experienced itching in your genital area? When did it start? Has it been treated? How?

5. Have you noticed any discharge from your vagina? If so, please describe its color, odor, and amount. When did you first notice it?

6. Have you had any vaginal bleeding aside from normal menstruation?

7. Do you have any pain, tenderness, or soreness in your pelvic area? Describe it (eg, dull, radiating, intermittent). When did it start? What makes the pain better or worse? Do you have associated symptoms of headache, vomiting, or diarrhea?

8. Have you had any surgery of the reproductive system? If so, what, when, and where?

9. Have you ever had an abnormal Pap smear? If so, when, and what treatment did you receive? Have you had follow-up Pap smears? When, and with what results?

Sexual Function

1. Are you able to be sexually aroused? Has this ability changed recently or over time?

2. Are you satisfied with your sexual experiences? If not, are you able to achieve orgasm?

Menstruation

1. What was the first day of your last period? How many days does your cycle usually run? Is this consistent from month to month?

2. How do you usually feel just before your period? How do you usually feel during your period? Do you use any self-care remedies?

3. How do you relieve cramps? Do you take medication? What do you take and how much?

Menopause

1. When did menopause begin for you?
2. What physical changes have you noticed?
3. Are you on estrogen therapy?
4. Have you had any vaginal bleeding since starting menopause?

Pregnancy

1. Have you ever been pregnant? If so, how many times?
2. Did you have any problems during pregnancy, delivery, or postpartum? If so, please describe.
3. Have you ever had a miscarriage? What were you told was the cause? Was surgery required?
4. Have you ever had an abortion? At how many weeks and by what method?
5. How has it been for you emotionally since the miscarriage/abortion?

Male and Female Clients

Fertility

1. Have you tried to have children? How long have you been trying?
2. *If client has been unable to conceive after 1 year*: How often do you have intercourse?
3. Have you ever sought professional help for fertility problems? If so, describe your experience.
4. Has an inability to conceive placed a strain on your relationship with your partner? How has it affected your relationship? How do you feel about this?

Sexual Practices

1. *If client is sexually active:* Are you in a mutually monogamous relationship? If not, how many sexual partners have you or your partner had over the last year?
2. Have you ever had a sexually transmitted disease? If yes, was it treated? Did you inform your partner? Did you have sex while you were infected? Did you use condoms?

3. Are you aware of having had any exposure to HIV? Describe the situation and how you feel you were exposed. What are your views on the potential for acquiring HIV?
4. Have you been tested for HIV? Once or routinely?

Self-Care

1. Do you check your genitals routinely? How often? *Male client:* Do you know how to perform a testicular self-exam? How often do you perform it and by what technique?
2. How often do you get a physical examination?
3. Are you using contraception? If so, what kind? Do you use it consistently? Would you like to know more about birth control?
4. How do you protect yourself from HIV and other sexually transmitted diseases?

Physical Assessment of the Male

- Gather the following equipment:

  culturette set   lubricant

  drape   penlight

  examination gloves
- Ask the client to empty bladder before the examination.
- Ask the client to remove any clothing below the waist.
- Review agency protocols before performing a detailed examination.
- Put on examination gloves. Change gloves during examination to prevent cross-contamination and exposure to body fluids.
- Culture any abnormal discharge.
- If client experiences an erection during the exam, explain that it is normal and has no sexual connotation, and then continue with a professional demeanor.

Assessment Techniques/ Normal Findings	Special Considerations

Inspection

1. Inspect the penis.

- Confirm that skin is loose over flaccid penis.
- Confirm that dorsal vein is midline on shaft.
- Confirm that glans is smooth and free of lesions, discharge, redness, or inflammation. Smegma is normal.

Discharge or lesions may indicate presence of infective diseases such as herpes, genital warts, or syphilis, or may indicate cancer. Culture any discharge and note consistency, color, and odor.

Alert!

Remember to change gloves as needed to prevent cross-contamination. Also, culture any abnormal discharge.

- For an uncircumcised client, either ask the client to pull back the foreskin or do so yourself, then gently move the foreskin back into place. Confirm smooth movement.
- Confirm that the urinary meatus is in the center of the penis tip.

Note *phimosis* or *paraphimosis*.

Referral

Seek immediate assistance if the foreskin cannot be retracted. Prolonged constriction of vessels can obstruct blood flow and lead to tissue damage or necrosis.

Note *epispadias, hypospadias,* or *urethral stricture.*

2. Inspect the scrotum.

- Ask the client to hold his penis up to fully expose the scrotum, or hold penis up on back of your nondominant hand. Confirm that scrotum is pearshaped, with left side hanging lower than right.

Appearance of flatness could suggest testicular abnormality. Swelling and inflammation could indicate *orchitis, epididymitis, scrotal edema, scrotal hernia,* or *testicular torsion,* as well as renal, cardiovascular, and other systemic disorders.

Assessment Techniques/ Normal Findings	Special Considerations
• If mass is detected, transilluminate the area in which the mass was palpated. Confirm that light shines through scrotum with red glow. The testicle appears as a nontransparent oval structure. Repeat with the other side and compare.	Note any area where light does not transilluminate—indicating a mass—which could be a *testicular tumor, spermatocele,* or other conditions.

3. Inspect the inguinal area.
Inspect the right and left inguinal areas with client breathing normally. Then have the client bear down, as if having bowel movement. Confirm flat appearance and even contour, free of lumps or masses.

Masses or lumps could be related to an inguinal hernia or cancer

Alert!
Some clients may not tolerate bearing down for more than a few seconds. Do not ask hypertensive clients to perform this maneuver.

Palpation

1. Palpate the penis.
• Place the glans between the thumb and forefinger and gently compress, allowing the meatus to gape open. Watch the client for nonverbal facial and body gestures that indicate pain. Confirm a pink, patent meatus, free of discharge.
• If urethritis is suspected, ask the client if he experiences itching and tenderness around the meatus and painful urination.
• Continue gentle palpation and compression up the entire penile shaft.

A pinpoint-size meatus could indicate urethral stricture.

Redness and edema around the glans and foreskin, eversion of urethral mucosa, and drainage are signs of urethritis. Note color, consistency, odor and amount of any discharge and obtain a specimen.

Profuse, thick, and purulent greenish-yellow discharge suggests gonorrhea.

Redness, edema, and discharge around the urethral opening indicate inflammation or infection higher up in urinary tract.

Note tenderness, lesions, masses, swelling, or nodules.

Assessment Techniques/ Normal Findings	Special Considerations

2. Palpate the scrotum.
Ask the client to hold penis up to expose scrotum. Gently palpate both scrotal sacs. Confirm that sacs are nontender, soft, and boggy, and that structures within sacs move easily.

Alert!
Do not pinch or squeeze any mass, lesion, or other structure.

Assess the shape, size, consistency, location, and mobility of any masses. If the client expresses pain, lift the scrotum; if pain is relieved, the client may have epididymitis. Note tenderness, swelling, masses, lesions, or nodules.

3. Palpate the testes.
With warm hands, approach each testis from bottom of the scrotal sac and gently rotate it between your thumb and fingertips. Confirm that each testis is nontender, oval-shaped, walnut-sized, smooth, elastic, and solid.

The *cremasteric reflex*—caused by cold hands, a cold room, or touch—could cause testicles to migrate upward temporarily.

4. Palpate the epididymes.
Slide fingertips to the posterior side of each testicle to find the epididymis, a small, crescent-shaped structure. Gently palpate. This should not cause pain.

In some clients, the epididymis can be palpated on the front surface.

5. Palpate the spermatic cord.
· Slide fingers up just above the testicle, feeling for a vertical, rope-like structure about 3 mm wide. Gently grasp it between your thumb and index finger without squeezing or pinching (Figure 12.1).

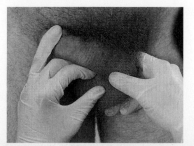

Figure 12.1   Palpating the spermatic cord.

Assessment Techniques/ Normal Findings	Special Considerations
• Using a gentle rotating motion, trace the cord up to the external inguinal ring. Confirm a thin, smooth, nontender, resilient feeling.	A hard, beaded, or nodular cord could indicate varicosity or a varicocele.

6. Palpate the inguinal region.

Alert!
This is a very sensitive, ticklish area. Use firm, deliberate movements and instruct the client to inform you of any pain or discomfort.

• Ask the client to shift weight to his left leg.
• Place right index finger in upper corner of the right scrotum, then slowly palpate the spermatic cord up and slightly to the client's left, allowing scrotal skin to fold over your index finger.
• Proceed to external ring of inguinal canal. Attempt to gently glide finger into the opening. If your finger is admitted, ask client to either cough or bear down, as you palpate for masses or lumps.

Alert!
If you cannot insert finger with gentle pressure, do not force into opening.

• Repeat in left inguinal area with the client's weight on the right leg and using your left index finger.

A bulge or mass could be an *inguinal hernia*. A *direct inguinal hernia* can be palpated in the area of the external ring; an *indirect inguinal hernia* is located deeper in the inguinal canal and can pass into the scrotum; a *femoral hernia* is commonly found in the right inguinal area near the inguinal ligament. Table 12.1 illustrates these three types of hernias.

Referral
An acute bulge with tenderness, pain, nausea, or vomiting may indicate a strangulated hernia. Help client lie down and get immediate medical assistance.

Table 12.1   Inguinal Hernias

Type of Hernia	Characteristics	Signs and Symptoms
Direct hernia Internal ring / External ring	• Extrusion of abdominal intestine into inguinal ring. • Bulging occurs in the area around the pubis. • Occurs much more commonly in men.	• Most often is painless. • Appears as a swelling. • During palpation, have the client cough. You will feel pressure against the side of your finger.
Indirect hernia Internal ring / External ring	• Abdominal intestine may remain within the inguinal canal or extrude past the external ring. • Most common type of hernia.	• Appears as a swelling. • During palpation, have the client cough. You will feel pressure against your fingertip.
Femoral hernia Femoral canal	• Located within the femoral canal. • Bulge occurs over the area of the femoral artery. The right femoral artery is affected more frequently than the left. • Lowest incidence of all three hernias.	• Palpable soft mass. • May not be painful; however, once strangulation occurs, pain is severe.

Assessment Techniques/ Normal Findings	Special Considerations

7. Palpate the inguinal lymph chain.

Using pads of your first three fingers, palpate inguinal lymph nodes. Confirm that nodes are nonpalpable (or palpable but less than 0.5 cm, spongy, movable, and nontender). Confirm that the area is nontender (Figure 12.2).

Assess if the node is larger than 0.5 cm or if multiple nodes are present. Tenderness suggests an infection of the scrotum, penis, or groin area.

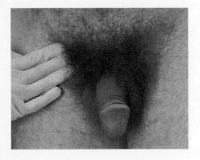

Figure 12.2 Palpating the inguinal lymph nodes.

8. Palpate the bulbourethral gland and the prostate gland.

· Ask the client to face the table and bend over at the waist, resting arms on table if desired. If the client cannot tolerate this position, he can lie with his left side on the table with both knees flexed.

· Lubricate your right index finger and tell the client you are going insert a finger into his rectum to palpate the prostate gland. Explain that it may cause him to feel as if he needs to have a bowel movement. Tell him to inform you immediately if the procedure causes pain.

Assessment Techniques/ Normal Findings	Special Considerations

- Place your index finger against the anal opening. Be sure your finger is slightly bent and not at a right angle to the buttocks. Apply gentle pressure and insert your bent finger into the anus. As the sphincter muscle tightens, stop insertion until the muscle relaxes. Then resume.

- Press right thumb gently against the perianal area. Palpate the bulbourethral gland by pressing the index finger gently toward thumb. Confirm absence of pain, tenderness, swelling, or masses (Figure 12.3).

Pain upon palpation could indicate an inflamed bulbourethral gland.

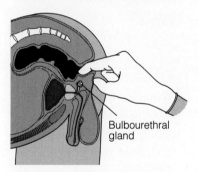

Bulbourethral gland

Figure 12.3   Palpating the bulbourethral gland.

- Release pressure between index finger and thumb, then continue to gently insert index finger. Palpate posterior surface of prostate gland. Confirm smooth, firm, possibly rubbery, nontender feel and that it extends no more than 1 cm into the rectal area (Figure 12.4).

Note tenderness, masses, nodules, hardness, or softness. Nodules are characteristic of prostate cancer, while tenderness indicates inflammation.

Assessment Techniques/ Normal Findings	Special Considerations

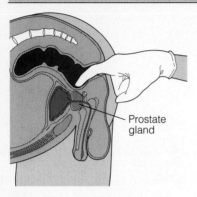

Prostate gland

Figure 12.4 Palpating the prostate gland.

Physical Assessment of the Female

- Gather the following equipment:

appropriate size speculum

bifid spatula

cotton-tipped applicators or cytobrush

culturette set

cytologic fixative for specimens

drape

examination gloves

examination gown

gooseneck lamp

hand-held mirror

lubricating jelly

prelabeled glass slides for specimens

receptacle for used speculum

sterile saline solution

- Ask the client to empty bladder and bowels before examination.
- Ask the client to remove clothing and put on an examination gown.
- Put on examination gloves. Change gloves during examination to prevent cross-contamination and exposure to body fluids.
- Culture any abnormal discharge.

Assessment Techniques/ Normal Findings	Special Considerations

1. Position the client.

Ask the client to lie on examination table. Assist her into lithotomy position and have her slide her hips as close as possible to the end of the table. Place her feet in the stirrups.

2. Inspect pubic hair.

• Confirm inverted triangle shape, with hair heavy over mons pubis and sparse over labia majora, perineum, and inner thighs.

Sparse hair pattern is common in Asians and elderly females, but may indicate delayed puberty.

• If client has complained of itching in pubic area, comb through pubic hair with two or three fingers. Confirm absence of crab lice.

Small, bluish-gray spots or nits at the base of pubic hairs or marks from persistent scratching indicate crab lice.

3. Inspect the labia majora.

• Confirm that labia majora are symmetric, and fuller and rounder in center, and that skin is smooth and intact.

Labia majora of elderly females may be thinner and wrinkled.

• Confirm absence of rashes, lesions, warts, vesicles, or ulcerations, and swelling or inflammation.

If drainage is found, note color, distribution, location, and characteristics.

Alert!

Remember to change gloves as needed to prevent cross-contamination. Also, culture any abnormal discharge.

A red rash with weepy, crusty lesions (often with scratches from itching) suggests *contact dermatitis*. *Genital warts* are raised, moist, cauliflower-shaped papules. Red, painful vesicles with localized swelling could indicate a *herpes* infection.

Swelling over red, inflamed, tender, and warm skin could indicate a Bartholin's gland abscess caused by gonorrhea.

Assessment Techniques/ Normal Findings	Special Considerations
4. Inspect the labia minora. Confirm that labia minora are smooth, pink, and moist. Observe for any redness or swelling. Note any bruises or torn skin.	Labia minora of elderly female may be drier and thinner. Redness and swelling indicate infective or inflammatory process. Bruises or torn skin suggest forceful intercourse or sexual abuse, especially in adolescents and children.
5. Inspect the clitoris. Place hand over the labia majora and separate with your thumb and index finger. Confirm that the clitoris is midline, about 1 cm long, full in center, smooth, and free of redness, lesions, and tears.	An elongated clitoris may indicate elevated testosterone levels and warrants referral to physician.
6. Inspect the urethral orifice. • Confirm that the urethral opening is midline, pink, smooth, slitlike, and patent. • Ask the client to cough, and check for a urine leak. • Inspect for any redness, inflammation, or discharge.	Urine leakage indicates stress incontinence and weakening of pelvic musculature. Redness, inflammation, or discharge indicate urinary tract infection.
7. Inspect the vaginal opening and perineum. Confirm that the vaginal opening is pink, round, and smooth or irregular.	

Palpation

1. Palpate the vaginal walls.
• Place your left hand above the labia majora and spread labia minora apart with thumb and index finger.

Assessment Techniques/ Normal Findings	Special Considerations

- With your right palm facing up, gently place right index finger at vaginal opening, then gently insert it into the vagina. Gently rotate finger counterclockwise, confirming rugated, consistent, and soft feel of the vaginal wall.

- Ask the client to bear down or cough, and check for bulging or protrusions.

Bulging or protrusions could indicate a prolapsed uterus, cystocele, or rectocele.

2. Palpate the urethra and Skene's glands.

- With right index finger, apply very gentle pressure upward against the vaginal wall. Stroke outward to milk Skene's glands (Figure 12.5).

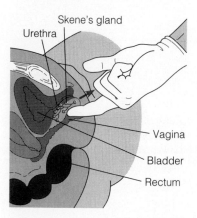

Figure 12.5   Palpating Skene's glands.

- Apply same upward/outward pressure on both sides of the urethra. Confirm absence of pain and discharge.

Discharge may indicate an infection such as gonorrhea. Obtain a culture.

Assessment Techniques/ Normal Findings	Special Considerations

2. Palpate the Bartholin's glands.

- With right index finger inserted in the vagina, gently squeeze the posterior region of labia majora between right index finger and right thumb (Figure 12.6).

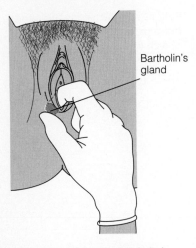

Bartholin's gland

Figure 12.6 Palpating Bartholin's glands.

- Perform this maneuver bilaterally, palpating both Bartholin's glands. Confirm absence of lumps, hardness, pain, or discharge.

Lumps, hardness, pain, or discharge suggest abscess and infection, possibly gonorrhea. Obtain a culture.

Inspection with a Speculum

Alert!

To ensure accuracy, make certain that the client has not douched within 24 hours before obtaining cervical and vaginal specimens.

If the client has vaginitis, delay speculum examination until treated unless this is the chief complaint and reason for the visit.

1. Select a speculum.

Select a proper size of speculum for the client and prewarm with a heating pad. Do not prewarm with water. Do not use gel lubricant.

Assessment Techniques/ Normal Findings	Special Considerations

2. Hold the speculum in your dominant hand.

Place index finger on top of blades, third finger on bottom of blades, and thumb just under thumbscrew.

3. Insert the speculum.

- With your nondominant hand, place index and middle fingers on the posterior vaginal opening and gently press downward.

- Turn the speculum blades obliquely. Place blades over your fingers at the vaginal opening and slowly insert the closed speculum at a 45-degree downward angle.

- Ask the client to bear down as you insert the speculum (to help relax the muscles). Once the speculum is inserted, withdraw fingers and turn speculum clockwise until blades are horizontal. Advance the blades at a 45-degree angle until they are completely inserted. This should not cause pain.

Alert!

If insertion causes client pain, stop immediately and reevaluate technique.

- Squeeze handle to open blades, sweep speculum upward until the cervix comes into view, and adjust the blades until the cervix is fully exposed between the blades.

- Tighten the thumbscrew.

Assessment Techniques/ Normal Findings	Special Considerations

4. Visualize the cervix.

- Confirm that the cervix is pink, moist, round, centrally positioned, and has a small opening in the center.

- Note any bluish coloring.

Bluish coloring is seen during the second month of pregnancy. Otherwise, bluish color indicates cyanosis.

- Confirm that secretions are clear and odorless.

Foul-smelling green discharge is associated with gonorrhea. White discharge indicates candidiasis. Frothy yellow-green discharge suggests trichomoniasis. Yellow discharge could indicate chlamydial infection. A creamy-gray to white, fishy-smelling discharge indicates bacterial vaginosis.

- Confirm that cervix is free from erosions, ulcerations, lacerations, and polyps.

Erosions are associated with carcinoma or infections. Ulcerations can be due to carcinoma, syphilis, and tuberculosis. *Nabothian cysts* are benign.

Obtaining a Pap Smear and Gonorrhea Culture

1. Perform an endocervical swab.

- Carefully insert saline-moistened, cotton-tipped applicator or cytobrush into cervical os, then rotate in a complete circle. Do not use force to insert.

If you cannot slip applicator into os, a tumor may be blocking the opening.

- Roll a thin coat across a slide labeled "endocervical" and spray or place in container with fixative.

Assessment Techniques/ Normal Findings	Special Considerations

2. Obtain a cervical scrape.

- Insert bifid end of bifid spatula into the vagina and advance the fingerlike projection of bifid end gently into os.

- With shorter end resting on outer ridge of cervix, rotate applicator one full turn clockwise (Figure 12.7). Do not rotate more than once, or counterclockwise.

If client has had a hysterectomy, obtain a scrape from the surgical stump.

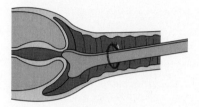

Figure 12.7   The cervical scrape.

- Spread thin smear across a slide labeled "cervical" from each side of the applicator and fix slide.

3. Obtain a vaginal pool sample. Insert paddle end of a spatula or saline-moistened cotton-tipped applicator into the fornix and gently rotate back and forth. Apply specimen to a slide labeled "vaginal" and fix slide.

4. Remove the speculum.

- Gently loosen the thumbscrew while holding handles securely. Slide speculum from the vaginal canal while slanting it from side to side.

Assessment Techniques/ Normal Findings	Special Considerations
• Confirm that vaginal mucosa is pink, consistent in texture, rugated, and nontender, and that discharge is thin or stringy, clear or opaque.	See descriptions of cervical discharge on page 158.
• Close speculum blades before complete removal.	

Bimanual Palpation

Stand at the end of the examination table, with the client remaining in the lithotomy position.

1. Palpate the cervix.

• Lubricate index and middle fingers of gloved dominant hand. Place your nondominant hand against the client's thigh, then insert lubricated fingers into the vaginal opening. Proceed downward at a 45-degree angle until you reach the cervix.

• Holding other fingers rounded inward toward palm, put thumb against mons pubis away from the clitoris.

• Palpate the cervix. Confirm smooth, firm feel.

• Gently try to move the cervix and confirm easy movement 1 to 2 cm in either direction.

Nodules, hardness, or lack of mobility suggest tumor. If the woman is pregnant, her cervix will be soft.

2. Palpate the fornices.

• Slip fingers into the fornices and palpate around the grooves.

• Confirm that mucosa of the vagina and cervix is smooth and nontender.

Assessment Techniques/ Normal Findings	Special Considerations

3. Palpate the uterus.

- With fingers still in the anterior fornix, place fingers of nondominant hand on the client's abdomen.

- Invaginate abdomen midway between umbilicus and symphysis pubis by pushing with fingertips downward toward the cervix (Figure 12.8).

Tenderness, masses, nodules, or bulging could indicate inflammation, infection, cysts, tumors, or wall prolapse. Note size, shape, consistency, and mobility of nodules or masses.

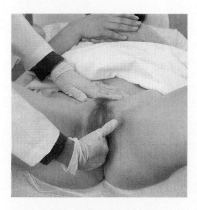

Figure 12.8 Palpating the uterus.

- Palpate the front wall of the uterus with hand inside the vagina and the back wall of the uterus with the other hand.

Inability to clearly differentiate uterine structures in an obese client may indicate need for an ultrasound study.

- Confirm normal position of the cervix in relation to position of the uterine body—uterus tilted slightly upward above the bladder with cervix tilted slightly forward. Normal variations are anteversion, midposition, and retroversion.

Anteflexion and retroflexion are abnormal variations.

Assessment Techniques/ Normal Findings	Special Considerations
• Move inner fingers to posterior fornix and gently raise the cervix up toward the outer hand. Palpate the front and back walls of uterus as it is sandwiched between your hands.	Further evaluate masses, tenderness, nodules, or bulging.

4. Palpate the ovaries.
• With fingers still in the vagina, position the outer hand on the left lower abdominal quadrant and slip vaginal fingers into the left lateral fornix.
• Push opposing fingers and hand toward each other, then use small circular motions to palpate the left ovary with intravaginal fingers (Figure 12.9).

Extreme tenderness, nodularity, and masses suggest inflammation, infection, cysts, malignancies, or tubal pregnancy.

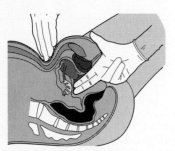

Figure 12.9 Palpating the ovaries.

• If palpable, the ovary should feel mobile, almond-shaped, smooth, firm, and nontender to slightly tender. Often, you will be unable to palpate ovaries, especially the right ovary.
• Slide intravaginal fingers to the right lateral fornix and outer hand to the lower right quadrant to palpate the right ovary.

Ovaries are difficult to palpate in obese females and in females who have been postmenopausal for more than 2.5 years.

Assessment Techniques/ Normal Findings	Special Considerations
• Confirm that uterine tubes are not palpable. • Remove hand from the vagina and put on new gloves.	Palpable uterine tubes suggest inflammation or other disease process.

5. Perform a rectovaginal exam.

- Lubricate gloved index and middle fingers of your dominant hand.
- Ask the client to bear down.
- Touch the client's thigh with your nondominant hand. Insert the gloved index finger into the vagina at a 45-degree downward slope and the middle finger into the rectum.
- Compress the rectovaginal septum between index and middle fingers and confirm that it is thin, smooth, and nontender.

Note tenderness, masses, nodules, bulging, and thickened areas.

- Place nondominant hand on the client's abdomen. While maintaining the position of the intravaginal hand, press inward and downward on the abdomen over the symphysis pubis.
- Palpate the posterior side of uterus with pad of rectal finger while continuing to press down on the abdomen. Confirm that the uterine wall is smooth and nontender (Figure 12.10).

Tenderness, masses, nodules, bulging, or thickened areas require further evaluation.

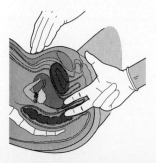

Figure 12.10 Rectovaginal palpation.

Nursing Diagnoses Commonly Associated with the Reproductive System

Altered sexuality patterns—state in which an individual expresses concern regarding his or her sexuality patterns

Sexual dysfunction—state in which an individual experiences a change in sexual function that is viewed as unsatisfying, unrewarding, or inadequate

Altered family processes

Altered growth and development

Body image disturbance

Fear

High risk for infection

Knowledge deficit

Rape-trauma syndrome

Rape-trauma syndrome—compound reaction

Common Reproductive System Alterations

Sexually Transmitted Diseases

Chancroid, chlamydia, genital herpes, genital warts, gonorrhea, syphilis, trichonomiasis.

Abnormal Cell Growth in Reproductive Organs

Female: cervical carcinoma, cervical polyps, myomas/fibroids, ovarian cancer, ovarian cysts, uterine cancer.

Male: penile carcinoma, prostate cancer, testicular cancer.

Inguinal Hernias

Direct hernia, femoral hernia, indirect hernia.

Reproductive System Client Education

Share the following information with the client.

Promoting a Healthy Reproductive System

- Maintain cleanliness and prevent infections by daily washing, keeping genitals dry, and changing underclothing daily.
- Seek counseling and support on issues of sexual function, sexual satisfaction, and sexual orientation.
- Seek health care for intense itching of genitals; genital rashes, warts, lesions, swelling, or discoloration; masses, lesions, or lumps, pain or tenderness in genital or abdominal area; changes in libido, painful intercourse, and persistent inability to achieve orgasm.
- *Female client:* Seek health care for bleeding problems and abnormal-colored or foul-smelling discharge from genitals.
- *Male client:* Seek health care for discharge from genitals, inability to achieve or maintain an erection, painful erection, or the inability to ejaculate.

Preventing Sexually Transmitted Diseases

- The risk of contracting an STD increases with the number of sexual partners.
- Other than abstinence, using condoms is the best way of preventing transmission of an STD. Additionally, a diaphragm, cervical cap, sponge, or spermicide offers some protection.
- Absence of symptoms does not mean absence of infection. If infection is suspected, evaluation is warranted.

Preventing Cancers of the Reproductive System

Understand the risk factors for cancer:

- Cervical cancer—multiple sexual partners, early and frequent sexual activity, STDs, smoking
- Uterine cancer—menstruation before age 12; no children or infertility; hypertension, diabetes mellitus, obesity; menopause that begins after age 50; long-term estrogen replacement therapy without progestin
- Ovarian cancer—family history of ovarian, breast, or uterine cancer; no children, infertility, or first pregnancy after age 30; repeated problems with regular ovulation
- Testicular cancer—possibly cryptorchidism, age of 20 to 40
- Prostatic cancer—possibly smoking, family history of prostatic cancer
- *Female client:* If sexually active now or in the past, have an annual pelvic examination with general physical examination. The Pap smear is effective in detecting cervical cancer and is partially effective as a screening tool for endometrial cancer. To date, no effective screening tool has been discovered for ovarian cancer.
- *Male client:* Perform testicular self-exam monthly, from adolescence.

Reproductive System Physical Assessment Summary

Physical Assessment of the Male

Inspection
1. Inspect the penis.
2. Inspect the scrotum.
3. Inspect the inguinal area.

Palpation
1. Palpate the penis.
2. Palpate the scrotum.
3. Palpate the testes.
4. Palpate the epididymes.
5. Palpate the spermatic cord.
6. Palpate the inguinal region.
7. Palpate the inguinal lymph chain.
8. Palpate the bulbourethral gland and the prostate gland.

Physical Assessment of the Female

Inspection
1. Position the client.
2. Inspect pubic hair.
3. Inspect the labia majora.
4. Inspect the labia minora.
5. Inspect the clitoris.
6. Inspect the urethral orifice.
7. Inspect the vaginal opening and perineum.

Palpation
1. Palpate the vaginal walls.
2. Palpate the urethra and Skene's glands.
3. Palpate the Bartholin's glands.

Inspection with a Speculum
1. Select a speculum.
2. Hold the speculum in your dominant hand.
3. Insert the speculum.
4. Visualize the cervix.

Obtaining a Pap Smear and Gonorrhea Culture
1. Perform an endocervical swab.
2. Obtain a cervical scrape.
3. Obtain a vaginal pool sample.
4. Remove the speculum.

Bimanual Palpation
1. Palpate the cervix.
2. Palpate the fornices.
3. Palpate the uterus.
4. Palpate the ovaries.
5. Perform a rectovaginal exam.

Chapter 13

Assessing the Peripheral Vascular and Lymphatic Systems

Focused Interview

Clients who have peripheral vascular changes may or may not be aware of any alteration in health. During the focused interview, gather information about the current health status of the client's peripheral vascular system, including the client's level of wellness, existing peripheral vascular problems, and interventions being implemented. Identifying pain and skin changes is particularly important.

1. Have you had or are you having any circulatory problems? If so, please describe the problem, including any treatment and resolution.
2. Have you or any family member had heart problems, respiratory disease, or diabetes?
3. Have you noticed any skin changes on your arms or legs? Describe. Have you noticed any swelling or shiny skin, particularly on your legs? Is the swelling in one leg or both? When did it start? Is the swelling worse at a certain time of day, or constant? What relieves the swelling?
4. Have you noticed any sores or ulcers on your legs? If so, is there any pain associated with the sores?
5. Have you noticed any temperature changes in your arms or legs, such as extreme coolness or heat?
6. Have you noticed numbness, tingling, or other changes in feeling in your legs?
7. Do you ever have leg pains or cramps? If so, describe the pain or cramp, the location, and when it most often occurs.
8. Do you smoke? If so, how long have you smoked? How much do you smoke daily?
9. What over-the-counter or prescription medications do you take?
10. Do you have swollen glands? If so, where are they? How long have

they been enlarged? Is there any related pain or redness? Have you
had other symptoms such as fever, fatigue, or bleeding?

11. Do you exercise regularly? If so, describe frequency, intensity, and
duration.

12. *Male clients:* Have you experienced any difficulty achieving an erection?

Physical Assessment

- Gather the following equipment:

  examination gown   sphygmomanometer

  examination gloves   stethoscope

- Ask client to remove all clothing except underwear and any tight
jewelry, and don the examination gown.
- During the assessment, you will be palpating body regions where
superficial nodes are located. Lymph nodes are small and normally
not palpable. Palpable nodes are usually enlarged and painful when
touched.
- Put on gloves if you notice open skin areas.

Assessment Techniques/ Normal Findings	Special Considerations

Blood Pressure

1. Take blood pressure in both arms with the client sitting.

2. Repeat Step 1 with the client supine.

3. Take blood pressure in both legs with the client supine. | If readings of more than 140 systolic or 90 diastolic are obtained, wait 30 minutes and repeat. If elevated readings remain, refer client to a physician.

Referral

Systolic reading below 90 and/or diastolic reading under 60 may be an early indication of shock, which requires immediate medical attention.

Assessment Techniques/ Normal Findings	Special Considerations

Arms

1. Assess hands.
Hold client's hands and note color of skin and nail bed and temperature and texture of skin. Note any lesions or swelling, or clubbing.

Flattening of nail base angle and clubbing suggests hypoxia in the extremities. A rounding of the fingertip, spongy nail, or blue discoloration of nail suggests chronic hypoxia.

2. Place both arms together and compare size.
Confirm similar size.

Edema in arms could indicate an obstruction of the lymphatic system.

3. Palpate radial pulses in both arms.
- Ask client to extend hand, palm up. Palpate with two fingers over lateral wrist.
- Note pulse rate, rhythm, amplitude, and symmetry. Grade amplitude according to the following four-point scale:

  4 = Bounding
  3 = Increased
  2 = Normal
  1 = Weak
  0 = Absent or nonpalpable

4. Palpate brachial pulses in both arms.
Ask client to extend arm. Palpate over brachial artery just superior to antecubital region (Figure 13.1). Note pulse rate, rhythm, amplitude, and symmetry. Grade amplitude on the four-point scale.

Use Doppler flowmeter positioned over patent artery if you have difficulty palpating pulses.

Assessment Techniques/ Normal Findings	Special Considerations

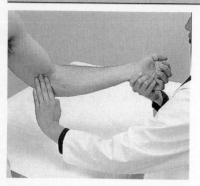

Figure 13.1 Palpating the brachial pulse.

5. Palpate epitrochlear lymph node in both arms.
Hold client's right hand in your right hand. With left hand, reach behind elbow to the groove between biceps and triceps. Note size and consistency of node, if palpable. Reverse for other arm.

An enlarged node may indicate an infection in the hand or forearm.

Legs

1. Inspect legs.
Confirm that skin color matches skin tone of rest of body and that hair growth is symmetric. Skin should be intact, with no lesions.

Pale leg skin indicates peripheral vessel constriction. Reddish skin indicates vessel dilation. Rusty discoloration over anterior tibial surface with skin intact is associated with decreased arterial circulation. If skin lesions or ulcerations are present, note size and location.

Referral
If blackened skin is found, refer client to physician immediately.

2. Compare size of legs.
Confirm symmetrical size. If unequal in size, measure circumference of bigger leg at widest point and compare with measurement of the same point on the other leg.

Size discrepancy could indicate edema from increased capillary pressure or lymph vessel obstruction. It could also indicate a blood clot in the deep vessels of the leg.

Assessment Techniques/ Normal Findings	Special Considerations
3. Palpate legs for temperature. Using dorsal surface of hands, palpate from feet up, noting discrepancies. Confirm that temperature is the same on both legs.	Cool skin may indicate peripheral vessel constriction. Warm skin may indicate peripheral vessel dilation. Temperature difference of feet could be a sign of arterial insufficiency.
4. Assess legs for presence of superficial veins.	
• Inspect legs with client sitting and legs dangling from examination table. Then ask client to elevate legs. Confirm that any bulges in veins disappear when legs are elevated. • Palpate veins for tenderness or inflammation.	*Varicosities* do not disappear when legs are elevated.
5. Palpate inguinal lymph nodes in both legs. Move client's gown aside over inguinal region. Palpate over top of medial thigh. Confirm that nodes—if palpable—are movable and nontender.	Lymph nodes larger than 1 cm or tender may indicate a leg infection.
6. Palpate femoral pulses in both legs.	Absence of femoral pulse could indicate an occluded artery.
• Ask client to bend knee out to the side. Palpate over femoral artery (inferior and medial to inguinal ligament). If necessary, place one hand on top of the other to locate pulse. • Note pulse rate, rhythm, and amplitude. Grade amplitude on the four-point scale. Note symmetry of pulses.	

Assessment Techniques/ Normal Findings	Special Considerations

7. Palpate popliteal pulses in both legs.

- Ask client to flex knee and relax leg. Palpate popliteal artery deep in popliteal fossa lateral to midline.
- If pulse is not found, ask client to lie prone and flex knee (Figure 13.2). Palpate deeply for pulse.

Absent popliteal pulse could indicate an occluded artery.

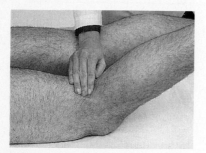

Figure 13.2 Palpating the popliteal pulse.

- Note pulse rate, rhythm, and amplitude. Grade amplitude on the four-point scale. Note symmetry of pulses.

8. Palpate dorsalis pedis pulses in both feet.

- Ask client to flex foot slightly. Using light pressure, palpate pulse lateral to extensor tendon of great toe (Figure 13.3).

Absence of dorsalis pedis pulse may not indicate occlusion because another artery may supply blood to that area of the foot.

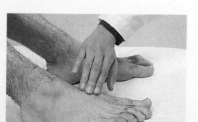

Figure 13.3 Palpating the dorsalis pedis pulse.

Assessment Techniques/ Normal Findings	Special Considerations

- Note pulse rate, rhythm, and amplitude. Grade amplitude on a four-point scale as above. Note symmetry of pulses.

9. Palpate posterior tibial pulses in both feet.
- Palpate posterior and tibial pulses by curving fingers around medial malleolus (Figure 13.4).

Absence of pulse could indicate an occluded artery.

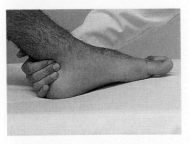

Figure 13.4 Palpating the posterior tibial pulse.

- Note pulse rate, rhythm, and amplitude. Grade amplitude on the four-point scale.

10. Check for edema of legs.
Press skin for at least 5 seconds over tibia, behind medial malleolus, and over dorsum of each foot. Look for depression in skin caused by pressure of fingers. If edema is present, grade on a scale of 1+ (mild) to 4+ (severe).

Pitting edema can be related to failure of the right side of the heart or an obstruction of the lymphatic system. Edema in one leg may indicate occlusion of a large vein in the leg.

Nursing Diagnoses Commonly Associated with the Peripheral Vascular and Lymphatic Systems

- **Activity intolerance**—state in which an individual has insufficient physiologic or psychologic energy to endure or complete required or desired daily activities

- **Altered tissue perfusion**—state in which an individual experiences a decrease in nutrition and oxygenation at the cellular level due to a deficit in capillary blood supply
- **Body image disturbance**
- **Disuse syndrome**
- **Fear**
- **High risk for injury**
- **Impaired mobility**
- **Impaired skin integrity**
- **Self-care deficit**

Common Peripheral Vascular and Lymphatic System Alterations

Arterial insufficiency, arterial aneurysm, deep vein thrombosis, Raynaud's disease, varicose veins, venous insufficiency.

Table 13.1, pp. 176–177, lists normal and abnormal pulses.

Peripheral Vascular and Lymphatic System Client Education

- Counsel clients with current alterations on how to prevent their health problems from worsening.
- Reduce the risk of heart attack and stroke by making lifestyle choices that can help reduce high blood pressure:

  Lose excess weight. Try to control weight though regular aerobic exercise and eating a low-fat diet.

  Reduce salt intake to help control hypertension.

  Consume no more than three alcoholic drinks per day; eliminating alcohol can lower blood pressure by more than 10 points.

  Quit smoking to help reduce the risk of stroke.

- For clients with venous or arterial insufficiency in lower limbs:

  Apply lotion to feet daily (not between toes).

  Inspect legs and feet daily for abrasions, blisters, or any trauma that could lead to infection.

  Wear support hose to promote venous return.

  If you have diabetes, control blood glucose to prevent vascular complications and avoid wearing garments that might inhibit circulation in the legs.

Peripheral Vascular and Lymphatic Systems Physical Assessment Summary

Blood Pressure

1. Take blood pressure in both arms with the client sitting.
2. Repeat Step 1 with the client supine.
3. Take blood pressure in both legs with the client supine.

Arms

1. Assess hands.
2. Place both arms together and compare size.
3. Palpate radial pulses in both arms.
4. Palpate both brachial pulses in both arms.
5. Palpate epitrochlear lymph node in both arms.

Legs

1. Inspect legs.
2. Compare size of legs.
3. Palpate legs for temperature.
4. Assess legs for presence of superficial veins.
5. Palpate inguinal lymph nodes in both legs.
6. Palpate femoral pulses in both legs.
7. Palpate popliteal pulses in both legs.
8. Palpate dorsalis pedis pulses in both feet.
9. Palpate posterior tibial pulses in both feet.
10. Check for edema of legs.

TABLE 13.1 Normal and Abnormal Pulses

Name of Pulse	Characteristics
Normal	• Regular, even in intensity
Absent	• No palpable pulse, no waveform
Weak/thready	• Intensity of pulse is +1 • May wax and wane • May be difficult to find
Bounding	• Intensity of pulse is +4 • Very easy to observe in arterial locations near surface of skin • Very easy to palpate and difficult to obliterate with pressure from fingertips
Biferiens	• Has two systolic peaks with a dip in between • Easier to detect in the carotid location • In the case of hypertrophic obstructive cardiomyopathy, only one systolic peak palpated, but waveform demonstrates double systolic peak
Pulsus alternans	• Alternating strong and weak pulses • Equal interval between each pulse
Pulsus bigeminus	• Alternating strong and weak pulses, but the weak pulse comes in early after the strong pulse
Pulsus paradoxus	• Reduced intensity of pulse during inspiration versus expiration
Water-Hammer, Corrigan's pulse	• Rapid systolic upstroke and no dicrotic notch secondary to rapid
Unequal	• Difference in intensity or amplitude between right and left pulses

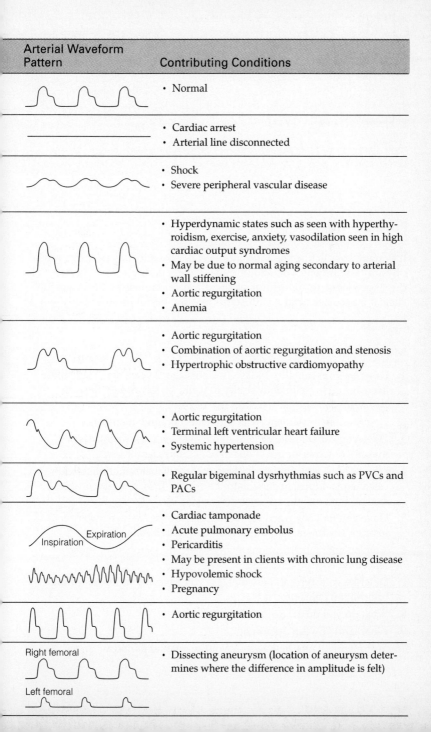

Arterial Waveform Pattern	Contributing Conditions
	• Normal
	• Cardiac arrest • Arterial line disconnected
	• Shock • Severe peripheral vascular disease
	• Hyperdynamic states such as seen with hyperthyroidism, exercise, anxiety, vasodilation seen in high cardiac output syndromes • May be due to normal aging secondary to arterial wall stiffening • Aortic regurgitation • Anemia
	• Aortic regurgitation • Combination of aortic regurgitation and stenosis • Hypertrophic obstructive cardiomyopathy
	• Aortic regurgitation • Terminal left ventricular heart failure • Systemic hypertension
	• Regular bigeminal dysrhythmias such as PVCs and PACs
	• Cardiac tamponade • Acute pulmonary embolus • Pericarditis • May be present in clients with chronic lung disease • Hypovolemic shock • Pregnancy
	• Aortic regurgitation
Right femoral / Left femoral	• Dissecting aneurysm (location of aneurysm determines where the difference in amplitude is felt)

Chapter 14

Assessing the Musculoskeletal System

Focused Interview

If you are conducting the musculoskeletal assessment as part of a total physical assessment, you should review your findings from the rest of the assessment to determine if there are relationships between the client's musculoskeletal health status and the health of other body systems.

Musculoskeletal System General Survey

1. Describe your mobility today, 2 months ago, 2 years ago. Have there been any changes in your ability to walk, sit, stand, eat, dress, or perform other simple activities free of pain?
2. Describe any musculoskeletal problems of family members.
3. Have you experienced any swelling, heat, redness, or stiffness in muscles or joints, or infections in bones, muscles, or joints?
4. Do you have any chronic diseases such as diabetes mellitus, sickle cell anemia, lupus, or rheumatoid arthritis? If so, describe progression and treatment of disease and impact on daily activities.
5. Have you had any fractures? If so, describe the frequency, cause, injuries, treatment, and impact on daily activities.
6. Are you taking medications such as steroids, estrogen, or muscle relaxants? Any other drugs?
7. Describe your typical daily diet. Do you have any problems eating or drinking dairy products?
8. What do you do for exercise?
9. What kind of work do you do?
10. *Premenopausal women:* Describe your menstrual periods.

Pain and Discomfort

1. *Clients with bone, muscle, or joint pain:* When did the pain begin? What were you doing when it began? What activities increase the pain? What activities decrease or eliminate the pain? Does it radiate? Do you experience unusual sensations, such as tingling, with the pain?
2. Do you experience constipation and/or abdominal distention?
3. Do you have difficulty breathing?

Physical Assessment

- Gather the following equipment:

  drape   examination light

  examination gloves   goniometer or tape measure

  examination gown

- Examine client in an orderly manner: head to toe, proximal to distal. Examine each joint with inspection first, then palpation. Assess range of motion (ROM), then assess muscle strength.
- When assessing ROM, demonstrate the ROM movement to the client while giving verbal instructions. Do not push the joint beyond its normal range, and stop if the client complains of discomfort. If ROM appears limited, measure the joint angle with a goniometer.
- To assess strength, ask the client to repeat the movements for ROM as you provide opposing force. The client should be able to perform movements against resistance, with equal muscle strength on both sides.
- You may need two or more sessions to complete an assessment of a client with compromised health status.
- Put on gloves if you notice open skin areas.

Assessment Techniques/ Normal Findings	Special Considerations
Temporomandibular Joint	
1. Inspect temporomandibular joint (TMJ) on both sides. Confirm that joints are symmetric and not swollen or painful.	Rounded protuberance indicates enlarged or swollen joint.

Assessment Techniques/ Normal Findings	Special Considerations

2. Palpate TMJ and jaw muscles.

- Palpate TMJ with index and middle fingers as client opens and closes mouth. Fingers should glide into shallow depression as mouth opens. Confirm smooth motion of mandible. Clicking is normal.

Findings of discomfort, swelling, crackling sounds, and limited jaw movement should be further evaluated.

- Have client clench teeth as you palpate masseter and temporalis muscles. Confirm that muscles are symmetric, firm, and nontender.

Swelling and tenderness suggest *arthritis* and *myofascial pain syndrome.*

3. Test ROM of TMJ.
Instruct client to perform the following movements:

- Open mouth as wide as possible. Confirm that mouth opens with ease to as much as 3 to 6 cm between upper and lower incisors.
- Hold mouth open slightly, then push out lower jaw. Return lower jaw to neutral position. Confirm that jaw protrudes and retracts with ease.
- Move jaw from side to side. Confirm lateral movement of 1 to 2 cm without deviation or dislocation.
- Close mouth. Confirm complete closing without pain or discomfort.

Suspect *TMJ dysfunction* if facial pain and limited jaw movement accompanies clicking sounds as jaw opens and closes.

Shoulders

1. Inspect shoulders.
With client facing you, verify symmetry and similar size of shoulders, clavicles, and scapula, anteriorly and posteriorly.

Swelling, deformity, atrophy, and malalignment, combined with limited motion, pain, and crepitus, suggest degenerative joint disease, traumatized joints, and inflammatory conditions.

Assessment Techniques/ Normal Findings	Special Considerations
2. Palpate shoulders and surrounding structures. • Begin at sternoclavicular joint and palpate laterally along clavicle to acromioclavicular joint. Then palpate downward into subacromial area and the greater tubercle of the humerus. • Confirm that these areas are firm and nontender, the shoulders are symmetric, and the scapula is level and symmetric.	**Referral** Shoulder pain without palpation or movement may result from insufficient circulation to the myocardium, which can be a precursor to a myocardial infarction. If client exhibits other symptoms, such as chest pain, indigestion, and cardiovascular changes, obtain medical assistance immediately. If client expresses discomfort, determine if pain is referred. Hiatal hernia and other conditions that increase abdominal pressure can cause shoulder pain.
3. Test ROM of shoulders. Instruct client to use both arms for the following movements: • Shrug shoulders by flexing forward and upward. • With elbows extended, raise arms forward and upward in an arc. Confirm 180-degree forward flexion. • Return arms to side. Keeping elbows extended, move arms backward as far as possible. Confirm extension of as much as 50 degrees. • Place backs of hands against back as close as possible to scapulae (internal rotation). • Clasp hands behind head (external rotation). • With elbows extended, swing arms out to sides in arcs, touching palms together above head. Confirm 180-degree abduction. • With elbows extended, swing arms toward body midline. Confirm adduction of as much as 50 degrees.	With rotator cuff tears, client will be unable to perform abduction without lifting or shrugging shoulders, pain, tenderness, and muscle atrophy.

Assessment Techniques/ Normal Findings	Special Considerations
4. Test strength of shoulder muscles. Have client repeat movements in Step 3 as you provide opposing force. Confirm that client can perform movements against resistance, with equal muscle strength on both sides.	Full resistance during shoulder shrug indicates adequate cranial nerve XI (spinal accessory) function.

Elbows

1. Inspect lateral and medial aspects of elbows. Support client's arms while inspecting. Verify symmetry.	Evaluate further if there is swelling, deformity, or malalignment. Elbow will appear deformed and forearm misaligned with subluxation.
2. Palpate lateral and medial aspects of olecranon process. Use thumb and middle fingers to palpate grooves on either side of olecranon process. Check for pain, thickening, swelling, or tenderness.	With inflammation, the grooves feel soft and spongy and surrounding tissue may be red, hot, and painful. *Rheumatoid arthriti*s may result in firm, nontender nodules (not attached to overlying skin) in olecranon bursa or along extensor surface of ulna. *Lateral epicondylitis* causes pain when client attempts to extend wrist against resistance. *Medial epicondylitis* causes pain when client attempts to flex wrist against resistance.
3. Test ROM of elbows. Instruct client to perform the following movements with one elbow, then the other: • Bend elbow by bringing forearm forward and touching fingers to shoulder. Confirm 160-degree flexion. • Straighten elbow. Confirm 0-degree extension.	

Assessment Techniques/ Normal Findings	Special Considerations

- Holding arm straight out, turn palm up and then down. Confirm 90-degree supination and pronation.
- Make certain that client can move elbow through a normal ROM without difficulty or discomfort.

4. Test strength of elbow muscles.
- Stabilize client's elbow with your nondominant hand while holding wrist with dominant hand.
- Have client flex and extend each elbow as you apply opposing force.
- Confirm that client can perform movements against resistance, with equal muscle strength on both sides.

Wrists and Hands

1. Inspect wrists and dorsum of hands for size, shape, symmetry, and color.
Confirm symmetry, absence of swelling and deformity, and color similar to the rest of the body.

Further evaluate redness, swelling, or deformity in joints.

2. Inspect palms.
Assess for rounded protuberance over thenar eminence.

Thenar atrophy is a finding associated with carpal tunnel syndrome, as well as with aging.

3. Palpate wrists and hands for temperature and texture.
Temperature should be warm and similar to the rest of the body. Skin should be smooth (knuckles may be rougher) and free of cuts.

Cool temperature in extremities may indicate compromised vascular function, which could influence muscle strength.

Assessment Techniques/ Normal Findings	Special Considerations

4. Palpate joints of wrists and hands.

- Keeping client's wrist straight, gently but firmly move your thumb over dorsum, with your fingers resting beneath the area you are palpating.
- Palpate sides of interphalangeal joints by pinching them gently between thumb and index finger. All joints should be firm and nontender, with no swelling.

A *ganglion* may require surgery.

5. Test ROM of wrists.

Instruct client to perform the following movements with one wrist, then the other:

- Straighten hand. Using wrist as pivot point, bring fingers backward as far as possible, then bend wrist downward. Confirm 70-degree hyperextension and 90-degree flexion.
- Turn palms down. Move hand laterally toward fifth finger and then medially toward thumb. Confirm 55-degree ulnar deviation and 20-degree radial deviation.
- Bend wrists downward and press backs of hands together (*Phalen's test*). Confirm 90-degree flexion without symptoms.

Most individuals with carpal tunnel syndrome will experience pain, tingling, and numbness that radiates to arm, shoulder, neck, or chest within a minute. If carpal tunnel syndrome is suspected, check for *Tinel's sign* by percussing lightly over median nerve in each wrist. If syndrome is present, client will feel numbness, tingling, and pain along median nerve.

Assessment Techniques/ Normal Findings	Special Considerations

6. Test ROM of hands and fingers.

Instruct client to perform the following movements:

- Make tight fist with each hand with fingers folded into palm and thumb across knuckles. Observe thumb flexion.
- Spread fingers apart, then back together. Confirm 20-degree abduction and full adduction.
- Point fingers downward toward forearm and then back as far as possible. Confirm 90-degree flexion and up to 30-degree hyperextension.
- Move thumb toward ulnar side of hand and then away from hand as far as possible. Touch thumb to tip of each finger and to base of little finger.

Inability to extend fourth and fifth fingers indicates Dupuytren's contracture.

Hips

1. Inspect positions of hips and legs.

Ask patient to lie with legs slightly apart and toes pointed toward ceiling.

External rotation of lower leg and foot is a classic sign of a fractured femur.

2. Palpate hip joints and upper thighs.

Confirm that hip joints are firm, stable, and nontender.

An unstable and deformed joint could indicate a fractured femur. Pain, tenderness, swelling, deformity, limited motion (especially internal rotation), and crepitus signal inflammatory or degenerative joint diseases.

Assessment Techniques/ Normal Findings	Special Considerations

3. Test ROM of hips.

Alert!

Clients who have undergone hip replacement should not perform these movements without permission of their physician.

Instruct client to perform the following movements:

- Raise each leg off bed or table with knee straight, keeping the other leg flat. Confirm 90-degree flexion.
- With knee flexed, raise each leg toward chest as far as possible. Confirm 120-degree hip flexion.
- Move each foot away from midline as knee moves toward midline. Confirm internal hip rotation of 40 degrees (Figure 14.1).

The client with a herniated disc will experience back and leg pain along the course of the sciatic nerve with this maneuver.

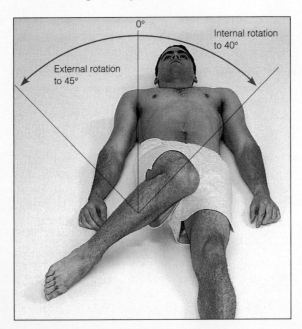

Figure 14.1 Internal and external hip rotation.

Assessment Techniques/ Normal Findings	Special Considerations

- Move each foot toward midline as knee moves away from midline. Confirm 45-degree external hip rotation (Figure 14.1).
- Move each leg away from midline, then as far as possible toward midline. Confirm 45-degree abduction and 30-degree adduction (Figure 14.2).

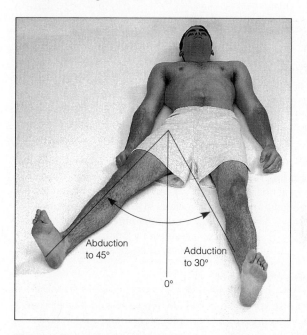

Figure 14.2   Abduction and adduction of the hip.

- Assist client to lie prone. With knee extended, raise leg as far as possible. Confirm 15-degree hyperextension of hips.

Assessment Techniques/ Normal Findings	Special Considerations

Knees

1. Inspect knees.
Ask client to lie supine. For each knee, confirm that the patella is centrally located, normal depressions along each side of the patella are sharp and distinct, and skin color is similar to that of surrounding areas.

Further evaluate swelling and signs of fluid in knee and surrounding structures. Fluid accumulates in suprapatellar bursa, prepatellar bursa, and other areas adjacent to patella with inflammation, trauma, or degenerative joint disease.

2. Inspect quadriceps muscles.

Atrophy occurs with disuse or chronic disorders.

3. Palpate each knee.
- Ask client to flex knee slightly. Beginning about 10 cm above patella, use your thumb, index, and middle fingers to palpate downward.
- Verify that the quadriceps muscle and surrounding soft tissue are firm and nontender. The suprapatellar bursa is usually not palpable.

Pain, swelling, thickening, or heat could indicate an *inflamed synovium*. Painless swelling frequently occurs in degenerative joint disease. Inflammation of the bursa results in a painful localized area of swelling, heat, and redness.

4. Palpate tibiofemoral joints of both knees.
With knee flexed, use your thumbs to palpate deeply along each side of tibia toward outer aspects of knee, then along lateral collateral ligament. Confirm that joint is firm and nontender.

Pain, tenderness, and other signs of inflammation could indicate degenerative joint disease, *synovitis,* or a *torn meniscus.* Bony ridges or prominences in outer aspects of joint occur with *osteoarthritis.*

5. Test ROM of knees.
- Instruct client to bend each knee against chest as far as possible and then return to extended position. Observe flexion.
- Have the client walk at a comfortable pace with relaxed gait.

Assessment Techniques/ Normal Findings	Special Considerations

6. Test strength of knee muscles.
Instruct client to flex and then extend each knee while you apply opposing force. Confirm that client can perform movements against resistance, with equal muscle strength on both sides.

7. Inspect knees while client stands.
Ask client to stand erect, holding back of chair if unsteady. Make certain knees are aligned with thighs and ankles.

Note *genu varum, genu valgum,* or *genu recurvatum.*

Ankles and Feet

1. Inspect ankles and feet with client sitting, standing, and walking.
Confirm that ankles and feet are symmetric and similar in color to the rest of the body, and that skin is smooth and unbroken. Feet and toes should be aligned with the long axis of the lower leg, with client's weight falling on the middle of the foot, and with no swelling present.

Evaluate further if *gouty arthritis, hallux valgus, hammertoe,* or *des planus* are present.

2. Palpate ankles.
Grasp heel of foot with fingers of both hands while palpating anterior and lateral aspects of ankle with your thumbs. Confirm firm, stable, and nontender joints.

Pain or discomfort on palpation and movement usually indicates degenerative joint disease.

3. Palpate length of calcaneal (Achilles) tendon at posterior ankle.
Confirm absence of pain, tenderness, and nodules.

Pain and tenderness along tendon could indicate tendinitis or bursitis. Small nodules are associated with rheumatoid arthritis.

Assessment Techniques/ Normal Findings	Special Considerations
4. Palpate metatarsophalangeal joints just below balls of feet. Confirm that joints are nontender.	Pain and discomfort suggests early involvement of rheumatoid arthritis. Acute inflammation of the first metatarsophalangeal joint suggests gout.
5. Palpate interphalangeal joints. Confirm that temperature is similar to the rest of the body.	Temperature in lower extremities that is significantly cooler than the rest of the body could indicate vascular insufficiency, which in turn may lead to musculoskeletal abnormalities.
	Pain, swelling, or tenderness could indicate inflammation or degenerative joint disease.
6. Test ROM of ankles and feet. Instruct client to perform the following movements with one foot and ankle, then the other: • Point foot toward nose. Confirm 20-degree dorsiflexion. • Point foot toward floor. Confirm 45-degree plantar flexion. • While stabilizing the client's ankle with one hand and heel with the other, ask client to point sole of foot outward then inward. Confirm 20-degree eversion and 30-degree inversion (Figure 14.3). • Curl toes downward. Observe flexion. • Spread toes as far apart as possible, then bring together again. Confirm ability to perform abduction and adduction.	Limited ROM and painful movement of foot and ankle without signs of inflammation suggest degenerative joint disease.

Assessment Techniques/ Normal Findings	Special Considerations

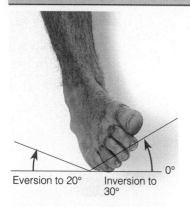

Eversion to 20°   Inversion to 30°   0°

Figure 14.3   Eversion and inversion of the ankles.

7. Test strength of ankle muscles.
Have client repeat dorsiflexion
and plantar flexion movements in
Step 6 as you provide opposing
force. Confirm that client can perform movements against resistance, with equal muscle strength
on both sides.

Spine

1. Inspect spine.
With client standing, check position and alignment of client's
spine from all sides:
• Confirm concave cervical and
lumbar curves and convex thoracic curve (Figure 14.4a).
• Imagine a vertical line from the
level of T1 to the gluteal cleft.
Confirm straight spine (Figure
14.4b).

Evaluate further with *kyphosis, lordosis, flattened lumbar curve, list,* or
scoliosis.

Assessment Techniques/ Normal Findings	Special Considerations

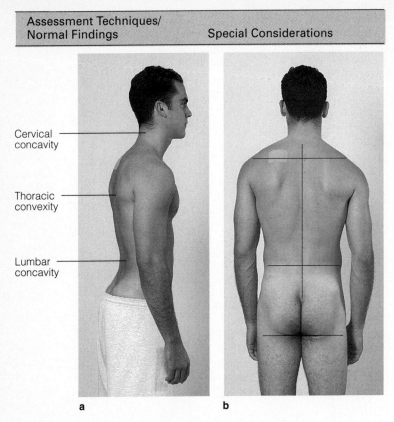

Cervical concavity

Thoracic convexity

Lumbar concavity

a   b

Figure 14.4 Lateral and posterior views of the normal spine.

• Imagine a horizontal line across the top of the scapulae. Confirm that scapulae are level and symmetric.	Lack of scapulae symmetry could indicate thoracic surgery or lung removal.
• Confirm level heights of iliac crests and gluteal folds.	
2. Palpate each vertebral process with thumb. Confirm aligned vertebral processes, uniform in size, firm, stable, and nontender.	If client is elderly, complains of pain or tenderness, and has restricted back movement, a compression fracture may be the cause.

Assessment Techniques/ Normal Findings	Special Considerations
3. Palpate muscles on neck and back. Verify that neck muscles are fully developed and symmetric, firm, smooth, and nontender.	Muscle spasms feel like hardened or knot-like formations. When they occur, client will complain of pain and restricted movement. They are associated with TMJ dysfunction or *spasmodic torticollis.*
4. Test ROM of cervical spine. Instruct client to perform the following movements: • Touch chest with chin. Confirm cervical spine flexion. • Look up toward ceiling. Confirm cervical spine hyperextension. • Attempt to touch each shoulder with ear, holding the shoulder level. Confirm cervical spine lateral bending. • Turn head as far as possible on each side. Confirm cervical spine rotation.	
5. Test ROM of thoracic and lumbar spine. Sitting or standing behind client, stabilize pelvis with your hands and instruct client to perform the following movements: • Bend sideways to the right and to the left. Confirm 35-degree right and left lateral flexion. • Bend forward and touch toes. Confirm that lumbar concavity disappears and back assumes C-shaped convexity with flexion. • Bend backward as far as is comfortable. Confirm 30-degree hyperextension. • Twist shoulders to left and right. Confirm 30-degree rotation.	Limited ROM, crepitation, or pain on movement in the joint require further evaluation. If client complains of sharp pain that begins in the lower back and radiates down leg, perform the straight-leg raising test: Keeping knee extended, raise client's leg until pain occurs, then dorsiflex client's foot. Record distribution and severity of pain and degree of leg elevation at the time pain occurs. Also record whether dorsiflexion increases pain. Pain with straight-leg raising may indicate a herniated disc.

Nursing Diagnoses Commonly Associated with the Musculoskeletal System

- **Activity intolerance**—related to immobility
- **Body-image disturbance**—related to musculoskeletal changes
- **High risk for disuse syndrome**—state in which an individual is at risk for deterioration of body systems as the result of prescribed or unavoidable inactivity
- **High risk for injury**—state in which an individual is at risk for injury as a result of environmental conditions interacting with the individual's adaptive and defensive resources
- **High risk for trauma**—accentuated risk of accidental tissue injury (eg, wound, burn, fracture)
- **Impaired physical mobility**—limitation of ability for independent physical movement

  Level I: Independently uses equipment or device

  Level II: Requires help from another person for assistance, supervision, or teaching

  Level III: Requires help from another person and equipment/device

  Level IV: Is dependent and does not participate in activity

- **Knowledge deficit**—inadequate information concerning self-care
- **Pain**—related to degeneration of soft tissue in the joints
- **Social isolation**—related to musculoskeletal changes

Common Musculoskeletal System Alterations

Bone Disorders

Ankylosing spondylitis (Marie-Strumpell disease), gout (gouty arthritis), osteitis deformans (Paget's disease), osteoarthritis, osteomyelitis, osteoporosis, rheumatoid arthritis.

Joint Disorders

Bunion, carpal tunnel syndrome, hallux valgus, hammertoe, lateral epicondylitis (tennis elbow), medial epicondylitis, temporomandibular joint (TMJ) syndrome.

Spinal Disorders

Kyphosis, list, lordosis, scoliosis.

Trauma-Induced Disorders

Dislocation, fracture, muscle sprain, muscle strain.

Musculoskeletal System Client Education

Following are some ideas for promoting the health of the musculoskeletal system.

Promoting Healthy Bones and Muscles

- Maintain a healthy weight.
- Do weight-bearing exercises (eg, walking or low-impact aerobics) at least three times a week.
- Eat a balanced diet that includes approximately 800 mg of calcium daily (to reduce risk of osteoporosis) and adequate protein and vitamins C and D (to maintain bone health and muscle tone and promote tissue healing).
- Avoid smoking, alcohol, and caffeine.

Preventing Injuries

- Use proper body mechanics, particularly when lifting objects.
- Maintain an erect posture.
- Maintain a safe environment—use night lights, bathtub and stair handrails, non-slip mats, and remove loose rugs.
- Wear properly fitting shoes with low, broad heels.
- Use seat belts and observe speed limits for motor vehicles.
- Wear glasses if needed.
- Use walkers, canes, and other assistive devices if needed.

Musculoskeletal System Physical Assessment Summary

Temporomandibular Joint

1. Inspect temporomandibular joint on both sides.
2. Palpate TMJ and jaw muscles.
3. Test ROM of TMJ.

Shoulders

1. Inspect shoulders.
2. Palpate shoulders and surrounding structures.
3. Test ROM of shoulders.
4. Test strength of shoulder muscles.

Elbows

1. Inspect lateral and medial aspects of elbows.
2. Palpate lateral and medial aspects of olecranon process.
3. Test ROM of elbows.
4. Test strength of elbow muscles.

Wrists and Hands

1. Inspect wrists and dorsum of hands for size, shape, symmetry, and color.
2. Inspect palms.
3. Palpate wrists and hands for temperature and texture.
4. Palpate joints of wrists and hands.
5. Test ROM of wrists.
6. Test ROM of hands and fingers.

Hips

1. Inspect positions of hips and legs.
2. Palpate hip joints and upper thighs.
3. Test ROM of hips.

Knees

1. Inspect knees.
2. Inspect quadriceps muscles.
3. Palpate each knee.
4. Palpate tibiofemoral joints of both knees.
5. Test ROM of knees.
6. Test strength of knee muscles.
7. Inspect knees while client stands.

Ankles and Feet

1. Inspect ankles and feet with client sitting, standing, and walking.
2. Palpate ankles.
3. Palpate length of calcaneal (Achilles) tendon at posterior ankle.
4. Palpate metatarsophalangeal joints just below balls of feet.
5. Palpate interphalangeal joints.
6. Test ROM of ankles and feet.
7. Test strength of ankle muscles.

Spine

1. Inspect spine.
2. Palpate each vertebral process with thumb.
3. Palpate muscles on neck and back.
4. Test ROM of cervical spine.
5. Test ROM of thoracic and lumbar spine.

Chapter 15

Assessing the Neurologic System

Focused Interview

During the health history, confirm information regarding a history of hypertension, stroke, meningitis, encephalitis, the use of alcohol and drugs, and prescribed medications. Before beginning the interview, review available data from diagnostic work. Be sure to assess a client's psychosocial health if the client is experiencing a neurologic deficit. Use the following questions to gather additional information on the neurologic system.

1. Ask client to complete the sentence: "A typical day in my life includes—"

2. What brings you here today?

3. Have you ever had an injury to your head or back? If so, what happened and when? What treatment did you receive? Do you experience related problems today?

4. Describe your memory. Do you need to write things down so you won't forget? Do you lose things easily? What did you do today before you came here?

5. Do you get headaches? If so, describe: sensation, location (same area or different), frequency, and severity (on a 1 to 10 scale). Are you able to function with the headaches? What do you think causes them? What do you do to relieve the pain? Does it work?

6. Do you have fainting spells? Do you have a history of seizures or convulsions? If so, when was the first seizure? When was your last? What happens immediately before the seizure? How do you feel afterwards? Have you been told about what your body does during the seizure? What medications do you take? Do you take them regularly?

7. Has your vision changed? Do you ever see two objects when you know there is just one? Can you see to the sides without turning

your head? When you go from a bright to dark area, do your eyes adjust rapidly?

8. Has your hearing changed? Have you noticed any ringing in the ears?

9. Has your ability to smell or taste changed?

10. Describe your balance. Do you notice tremors? Can you bend down, pick up a straight pin, and stand upright again? Do you drop, spill, or knock things over, or trip easily? If so, how long have you noticed the symptoms? Are the symptoms continuous? Getting worse? What do you do to control or limit the clumsiness?

11. Do you have any pain? If so, where? When did it begin? Is it constant or intermittent? What relieves or decreases the pain? What increases the pain? Does it interfere with your daily activities? How does it feel (sharp, burning, stabbing, etc.)? Rate the pain on a 1 to 10 scale, with 10 being the most severe.

12. Are you being or have you been exposed to insecticides, organic solvents, lead, toxic wastes, or other environmental hazards? If so, what, when, and for how long? What treatments have you had? Do you experience related problems today?

Physical Assessment

- Gather the following equipment:

applicator	printed material
cup of water	Snellen chart
drape	sterile cotton balls
examination gloves	sterile needle
examination gown	stethoscope
objects to touch (eg, paper clip, safety pin, coins)	substances to smell (eg, coffee, vanilla, perfume)
ophthalmoscope	tongue blade
penlight	tuning fork
percussion hammer	

- Ask client to remove all clothing except underwear, and don examination gown.
- Explain all procedures to the client, keeping in mind that a client with a neurologic deficit may require a more detailed explanation and more time to respond to a question or direction.
- Use universal precautions throughout the assessment.
- Work in an organized manner, assessing mental status, cranial nerves, motor functions, sensory function, then reflexes.

Assessment Techniques/ Normal Findings	Special Considerations

Mental Status

Assess the client's speech, sensorium, memory, ability to do calculations, and ability to think abstractly. Observe the client's hygiene, grooming, posture, body language, gait, facial expressions, and ability to follow directions. See Chapter 2 for specific questions to ask when assessing psychological well-being.

Cranial Nerves

1. Test olfactory nerve (CN I). *not tested during exam*
Ask client to close both eyes and close one naris. Place a familiar odor under open naris (eg, coffee, vanilla, perfume). Ask client to sniff and identify odor. Repeat with other naris.

Anosmia may be due to cranial nerve dysfunction, a cold, rhinitis, zinc deficiency, or genetics. A unilateral change in this sense may be indicative of a brain tumor.

2. Test optic nerve (CN II).
- Test near vision by asking client to read printed material. Observe distance of material from face and position of head.
- Use Snellen chart to test distant vision and color.
- Use ophthalmoscope to inspect fundus. Note color and shape of optic disc.

Swelling of the optic nerve as it enters the retina indicates *papilledema*, a symptom of increased intracranial pressure. It may indicate a brain tumor or intracranial hemorrhage.

Referral
If intracranial hemorrhage is suspected, immediate medical attention is required.

A change in optic disc color and decreased visual acuity can indicate MS or a brain tumor.

3. Test oculomotor, trochlear, and abducens nerves (CN III, IV, and VI).
Perform following tests (detailed descriptions appear in Chapter 6):
- Six cardinal points of gaze
- Direct and consensual pupillary reaction to light

Pathologic conditions include *nystagmus* (constant involuntary movement of the eye), *strabismus* (deviation in muscular coordination), *diplopia* (double vision), or *ptosis* of the upper lid (dropped lid related to muscle weakness).

Assessment Techniques/ Normal Findings	Special Considerations
• Convergence and accommodation of eyes	
4. Test trigeminal nerve (CN V). Test sensory function: Ask client to close eyes. Touch face with wisp of cotton and ask client to say "now" every time cotton is felt. Repeat test using sharp and dull stimuli, using random pattern. Assess all three nerve branches.	Document any loss of sensation, pain, or fasciculation.
Test corneal reflex: Have clients with contacts remove lenses. Ask client to look straight ahead. Touch cornea from side with a wisp of cotton. Confirm that client blinks.	Clients who wear contact lenses often have decreased or absent reflex.
Test trigeminal nerve motor function: Ask client to clench teeth tightly. Bilaterally palpate masseter and temporalis muscles to assess muscle strength. Ask client to open and close mouth several times. Observe for symmetry of mandible movement without deviation from midline.	Muscle pain, spasms, and deviation of mandible with movement can indicate myofascial pain dysfunction.
5. Test facial nerve (CN VII). Ask client to perform several functions such as smile, close both eyes, puff cheeks, frown, and raise eyebrows. Confirm symmetry of facial movements.	Asymmetry or muscle weakness (such as eyelid drooping or changes in nasolabial folds) may indicate nerve damage. Inability to perform motor tasks could indicate a lower or upper motor neuron disease.
6. Test vestibulocochlear nerve (CN VIII). Perform Weber test and Rinne test (discussed previously in Chapter 6).	Tinnitus and deafness are associated with the cochlear branch of the nerve; vertigo is associated with the vestibular portion.

Assessment Techniques/ Normal Findings	Special Considerations

7. Test glossopharyngeal and vagus nerves (CN IX and X).
Test motor activity:
Ask client to open mouth. Depress tongue with tongue blade and ask client to say "Ah." Confirm that soft palate rises and uvula remains in midline.

Unilateral palate and uvula movement indicate disease of nerve on opposite side.

Test gag reflex:
Explain to the client that you are going to lightly touch the throat with an applicator. Touch posterior wall of pharynx with applicator. Observe pharyngeal movement.

Referral
Clients with diminished or absent gag reflex have increased potential for aspiration and need medical evaluation.

Test motor activity of pharynx:
Ask client to drink water and describe ease or difficulty of swallowing. Note quality of voice or hoarseness when client speaks.

Difficulty with swallowing could be related to cranial nerve disease.

Voice changes could indicate lesions, paralysis, or other conditions.

8. Test the accessory nerve (CN XI).
Test trapezius muscle:
Ask client to shrug shoulders. Observe equality of shoulders, symmetry of action, and lack of fasciculations.

Note muscle weakness, muscle atrophy, fasciculations, uneven shoulders, and chin raising following flexion.

Test sternocleidomastoid muscle:
Ask client to turn head to the right and then to the left. Ask client to try to touch right ear to right shoulder without raising shoulder. Repeat on left side. Observe ease of movement and degree of range of motion.

Assessment Techniques/ Normal Findings	Special Considerations
9. Test the hypoglossal nerve (CN XII). Ask client to protrude and then retract tongue. Ask client to protrude tongue and move to the right and then to the left. Note ease and equality of movement.	Note atrophy, tremors, and paralysis. Ipsilateral paralysis demonstrates deviation and atrophy of involved side.

Motor Function

Alert!

Be prepared to support and protect client to prevent accident, injury, or fall.

1. Assess client's gait and balance. • Ask client to walk in the following ways: Across room and back Heel-to-toe for several yards On toes On heels • Observe posture. Is it stiff or relaxed? • Note equality of steps, walking pace, position and coordination of arms when walking, and ability to maintain balance with all activities.	Gait change could indicate drug or alcohol intoxication, motor neuron weakness, or muscle weakness.

2. Perform Romberg test.

Alert!

Stand next to client to prevent falls.

Ask client to stand with feet together, arms at side, and eyes open. Observe for swaying. Ask client to close eyes while maintaining position. Confirm only slight increase in swaying with eyes closed.	Greatly increased swaying or falling with eyes closed could indicate disease of posterior columns of spinal cord. When eyes are open, client will be able to maintain the position.

Assessment Techniques/ Normal Findings	Special Considerations
3. Assess client's ability to perform rapid alternating action. • Ask client to perform the following actions: Place hands palms down on thighs Turn hands palms up Return hands palms down Alternate palms-up/palms-down movement at a faster pace • Test one side at a time if a deficit is suspected. Observe rhythm, rate, and smoothness of movements.	Inability to perform this action could indicate upper motor neuron weakness.

Sensory Function

Alert!

Stop assessment if client tires during procedures, and continue at a later time. Be sure to test corresponding body parts. Use the distal-to-proximal approach along extremities. When client describes sensations accurately at a distal point, you do not need to proceed to a more proximal point. If deficit is detected at a distal point, proceed to proximal points while attempting to map specific area of deficit. Repeat testing to determine accuracy in areas of deficits.

Remember always to ask the client to describe the stimulus and location; do not suggest. In order to gain client understanding, you may need to demonstrate what you will do. Have client keep eyes closed during testing.

Assessment Techniques/ Normal Findings	Special Considerations
1. Assess client's ability to identify light touch. Touch various parts of the body (feet, arms, abdomen, face) with a wisp of cotton at random. Ask client to say "yes" or "now" when stimulus is perceived. Test corresponding dermatomes.	Note anesthesia, hyperesthesia, or hypesthesia.
2. Assess client's ability to distinguish difference between sharp and dull. Using a sterile safety pin, touch client with the sharp end and then the blunt end. Ask client to say "sharp" or "dull" to indicate sensation. Randomly alternate between sharp and dull stimulation. Test corresponding body parts.	Note analgesia or hypalgesia.
3. Assess client's ability to feel vibrations. Set turning fork in motion and place on bony parts of the body—toes, ankle, knee, iliac crest, spinal process, fingers, sternum, wrists, elbows. Ask client to say "now" when vibration is perceived and "stop" when it is no longer felt. If client's perception is accurate when you test the most distal aspects, end the test.	Loss of vibration sense can indicate a neuropathy associated with aging, diabetes, intoxication, or disease of the posterior column.
4. Test stereognosis, the ability to identify an object without seeing it. Ask client to close both eyes. Place common objects such as safety pins, paper clips, and different coins in each of the client's hands and ask client to identify. Test each object independently.	Inability to identify a familiar object could indicate cortical disease.

Assessment Techniques/ Normal Findings	Special Considerations

Reflexes

The client should be sitting or supine, with limbs placed so muscles are partially stretched. Hold the handle of the reflex hammer in your dominant hand between your thumb and index finger. Use your wrist to generate a brisk, direct, smooth arc for stimulation. Stimulate the reflex arc with a brisk tap to the tendon. After striking tendon, remove hammer immediately.

Evaluate response on 0 to 4+ scale:

0 = no response
1+= diminished
2+= normal
3+= brisk, above normal
4+= hyperactive
Repeat test for 0 and 1+ responses.

Absent or diminished reflexes may indicate neuromuscular disease, spinal cord injury, or lower motor neuron disease. Hyperactive reflexes may indicate upper motor neuron disease. Clonus confirms upper motor neuron disease.

1. Assess biceps reflex (C5, C6).

• Support client's lower arm with your nondominant hand. Ask client to position arm slightly flexed at elbow and palm up.
• Place thumb of your nondominant hand over biceps tendon, then briskly tap thumb with reflex hammer (Figure 15.1).

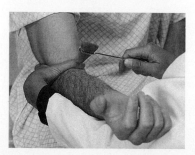

Figure 15.1   Testing the biceps reflex.

Assessment Techniques/ Normal Findings	Special Considerations

- Confirm contraction of biceps muscle and slight flexion of forearm. Repeat with the other arm.

2. Assess triceps reflex (C6, C7).
- Support client's elbow with your nondominant hand.
- Sharply percuss tendon just above olecranon process with reflex hammer (Figure 15.2).

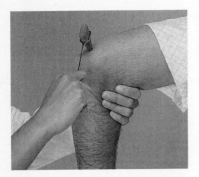

Figure 15.2 Testing the triceps reflex.

- Confirm contraction of triceps muscle with extension of lower arm. Repeat with the other arm.

3. Assess brachioradialis reflex (C5, C6).
- Position client's arm so elbow is flexed and hand is resting on lap with palm down.
- Briskly strike tendon toward radius about 5 to 7 cm above wrist with reflex hammer (Figure 15.3).

Assessment Techniques/ Normal Findings	Special Considerations

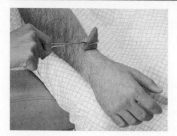

Figure 15.3   Testing the brachiora-dialis reflex.

- Confirm flexion of lower arm and supination of hand. Repeat with other arm.

4. Assess patellar reflex (L2, L3, L4). Flex leg at knee. Palpate patella to locate patellar tendon inferior to patella. Briskly strike tendon with reflex hammer. Confirm extension of lower leg and contraction of quadriceps muscle. Repeat with the other leg.

5. Assess Achilles tendon reflex (S1).
- Flex leg at knee. Dorsiflex foot and hold heel lightly in your nondominant hand.
- Strike Achilles tendon with reflex hammer (Figure 15.4).

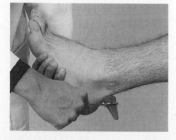

Figure 15.4   Testing the Achilles tendon reflex.

Assessment Techniques/ Normal Findings	Special Considerations
• Confirm plantar flexion of foot—heel will jump from hand. Repeat with the other leg.	
6. Assess plantar reflex (L5, S1). Position leg with slight degree of external rotation at hip. Stimulate sole of foot with wooden tongue blade from heel to ball of foot on lateral aspect, then across ball of foot to great toe. Confirm plantar flexion, with toes curling toward sole of foot. Repeat with the other foot.	A *Babinski response*, fanning of the toes with the great toe pointing toward the dorsum of the foot, is abnormal in adults and may indicate upper motor neuron disease.
7. Assess abdominal reflexes (T8, T9, T10 for upper and T10, T11, T12 for lower). Briskly stroke abdomen from lateral aspect toward umbilicus with applicator or tongue blade. Confirm muscular contraction and movement of umbilicus toward stimulus. Repeat in the other three quadrants of the abdomen.	Obesity and upper and lower motor neuron disease can diminish response.

Additional Assessment Technique

1. Evaluate level of consciousness with Glasgow coma scale. Figure 15.5 illustrates the scale.	**Referral** Client experiencing any loss of consciousness needs immediate medical intervention.

GLASGOW COMA SCALE
BEST EYE-OPENING RESPONSE 4 = Spontaneously 3 = To speech 2 = To pain 1 = No response **(Record "C" if eyes closed by swelling)**
BEST MOTOR RESPONSE to painful stimuli 6 = Obeys verbal command 5 = Localizes pain 4 = Flexion—withdrawal 3 = Flexion—abnormal 2 = Extension—abnormal 1 = No response **(Record best upper limb response)**
BEST VERBAL RESPONSE 5 = Oriented X 3 4 = Conversation—confused 3 = Speech—inappropriate 2 = Sounds—incomprehensible 1 = No response **(Record "E" if endotracheal tube in place,** **"T" if tracheostomy tube in place)**

Figure 15.5   Glasgow coma scale.

Nursing Diagnoses Commonly Associated with the Neurologic System

- **Altered thought process**—state in which individual experiences an impairment in cognitive operations, such as conscious thought, reality orientation, problem solving, and judgment. These impairments are a result of mental/personality or chronic organic disorders that may be exacerbated by situational crises.

- **Impaired verbal communication**—state in which an individual experiences a decreased or absent ability to use or understand language in human interaction
- **Impaired physical mobility**
- **Sensory/perceptual alterations**

Common Neurologic System Alterations

Gait

Ataxic gait, festination gait, scissors gait, steppage gait.

Movement

Athetoid movement, dystonia, fasciculation, myoclonus, tic, tremor.

Neurologic System Client Education

Explain that because many neurologic problems or disease processes can cause a permanent, nonreversible deficit, the focus must be on prevention rather than cure.

Safety

- Use safety equipment at work and during recreation.
- Use seat belts when driving. Use car seats for babies and young children.
- Control use and avoid misuse of firearms, drugs, and alcohol.
- Follow directions for medications, and become familiar with side effects.

Promoting General Health

- Prevent repeated systemic viral and bacterial infections by keeping your immune system healthy. Maintain your health with a nutritious diet, vitamin and nutritional supplements, rest, and regular exercise.
- Keep stress at a minimum by practicing stress-reduction techniques and developing effective coping strategies.
- Use proper body mechanics in all daily activities.

Neurologic System Physical Assessment Summary

Mental Status

Cranial Nerves

1. Test olfactory nerve (CN I).
2. Test optic nerve (CN II).
3. Test oculomotor, trochlear, and abducens nerves (CN III, IV, and VI).
4. Test trigeminal nerve (CN V).
5. Test facial nerve (CN VII).
6. Test vestibulocochlear nerve (CN VIII).
7. Test glossopharyngeal and vagus nerves (CN IX and X).
8. Test the accessory nerve (CN XI).
9. Test the hypoglossal nerve (CN XII).

Motor Function

1. Assess client's gait and balance.
2. Perform Romberg test.
3. Assess client's ability to perform rapid alternating action.

Sensory Function

1. Assess client's ability to identify light touch.
2. Assess client's ability to distinguish difference between sharp and dull.
3. Assess client's ability to feel vibrations.
4. Test stereognosis, the ability to identify an object without seeing it.

Reflexes

1. Assess biceps reflex (C5, C6).
2. Assess triceps reflex (C6, C7).
3. Assess brachioradialis reflex (C5, C6).
4. Assess patellar reflex (L2, L3, L4).
5. Assess Achilles tendon reflex (S1).
6. Assess plantar reflex (L5, S1).
7. Assess abdominal reflexes (T8, T9, T10 for upper and T10, T11, T12 for lower).

Additional Assessment Technique

1. Evaluate level of consciousness with Glasgow coma scale.

Chapter 16

Assessing Infants, Children, and Adolescents

Focused Interview

The history and physical assessment of the infant, child, or adolescent incorporates many elements of the adult history and assessment. However, children are not simply smaller versions of adults. Before continuing, you may want to review the anatomy and physiology of the healthy child and developmental tasks associated with the various stages of childhood.

Interviewing the Parent or Caregiver

- When taking the history of an infant or young child, gather most of the data from the parent or other caregiver.
- Do not assume that an adult accompanying a child is the child's parent. Always clarify the relationship to the child.
- If the child is seriously ill, you may need to begin interventions before you are able to complete the entire health history.

Interviewing the Child or Adolescent

- From about 5 years, a child will be able to respond meaningfully to questions about his or her health or illness. You may want to interview the older child alone, especially in cases where the child seems embarrassed, sullen, or confused.
- Be patient with adolescent clients who may have difficulty confiding in adults. You may find that beginning the interview by chatting about the client's school, social life, hobbies, sports activities, or job might help establish a trusting relationship.
- Respect the confidentiality of adolescents who are seeking health care on their own. Follow state laws and institutional guidelines for parental notification, always including the adolescent in the notification process.

Birth History

1. Describe the pregnancy (parity, problems, length of pregnancy, diet, weight gain, use of medications, illicit drugs, tobacco, and alcohol).
2. Describe the labor (course and duration, use of analgesia and anesthesia, obstetric procedures, type of birth, birth weight, Apgar scores, any medical problems).
3. Describe the postnatal period (problems in the hospital or after discharge, including feeding and sleeping problems, colic, diarrhea, postnatal depression, family problems).

Growth and Development

1. At what age did the child first (a) hold the head erect? (b) roll over? (c) sit up independently? (d) walk alone? (e) say words with meaning? (f) speak in sentences? (g) tie shoes? (h) dress without help? (i) get first tooth? (j) complete toilet training?
2. Do you believe that the child's development has been normal? Why or why not? How do you think the child's development compares with that of siblings or other children of the same age?

Psychosocial Health

1. Describe the child's typical day (note routine and structure, environment, amount of stimulation or deprivation).
2. *For older children and adolescents:* Describe a typical school day (note sleep patterns, stress level, extracurricular activities, employment, self-care, personal goals, family coping).
3. *For older children and adolescents:* How much alcohol do you consume each day? How many cigarettes do you smoke each day? Describe your typical daily diet. How much water do you drink each day?
4. *For adolescents:* Describe your present level of sexual activity.

Physical Assessment

- Gather the following equipment:

  centimeter measuring tape

  drape

  examination gloves

  examination gown

  ophthalmoscope

  otoscope with pneumatic bulb and ear pieces of various sizes

  sphygmomanometer and blood pressure cuff of appropriate size

  stethoscope

- Before beginning the assessment, encourage the toilet-trained child to void to decrease discomfort. When examining infants, leave the diaper on except when weighing or examining the perineum.
- Permit the young child to remain on the parent's lap for as much of the examination as possible.
- The most accurate assessment is obtained from the quiet child. Anxiety and crying alter vital signs, diminish the accuracy of lung and heart auscultation, and make abdominal palpation more difficult.
- Approach the physical assessment in a systematic manner, varying the sequence of the examination according to the child's age and degree of cooperation. Take advantage of quiet moments to listen to the heart and lungs. Postpone part of the assessment that the child may perceive as threatening until the end.
- Put on gloves to examine mucous membranes and to assess skin lesions, wounds, or any areas with blood, drainage, or body fluids.

Assessment Techniques/ Normal Findings	Special Considerations

General Appearance and Mental Status

1. Observe physical appearance, body structure, mobility, and behavior.	Obvious abnormalities, limitations of movement, behavior inappropriate for age, or poor hygiene may indicate the need for further investigation or parent and child education.
2. Observe interaction between child and parents. How does the parent hold the infant? Does the parent seem to be reading the infant's cues? Are the parent's expectations appropriate for the age of the child? How do the parent and child relate to each other?	Lack of attachment may be indicated when the parent holds the infant facing away, avoids eye contact with the infant, or fails to read infant's cues.
	Expecting a young child to sit quietly indicates a knowledge deficit of normal child development.
	An extremely negative or hostile interaction may indicate a disturbed parent-child relationship; intervention and referral are required.

Assessment Techniques/ Normal Findings	Special Considerations

3. Listen to the child's speech.
Note articulation, quantity, and organization of child's speech, as well as the child's thought processes. Can the older infant or toddler name objects or significant others? Can the preschool child ask and answer questions? Are the older children and adolescents able to contribute to the health history and answer age-appropriate questions?

Speech should be understandable by about three years of age. Speech delay or articulation problems in older infants or toddlers may indicate hearing deficit, lack of environmental stimulation, a bilingual environment, or generalized developmental delay.

Articulation problems in older children may indicate hearing deficit, learning disability, or language problem related to a bilingual environment.

Growth and Development

1. Obtain accurate height and weight measurements.
Plot the measurements on an age- and gender-appropriate growth chart. Both height and weight measurements should fall in approximately the same percentile. Try to obtain serial measurements, which provide a more accurate assessment of rate of growth.

Great discrepancies between height and weight percentile require further evaluation.

Low weight for height may indicate inadequate nutrition, cardiac problems, renal problems, or chronic systemic disease.

High weight for height may indicate overnutrition or a metabolic problem.

2. Measure the head circumference of children under 2 years of age.
Place the tape measure around the head just above the eyebrows and the ear pinna and around the most prominent area of the occiput. Plot the measurements on an appropriate growth chart.

A single head circumference measurement that falls above the 95th percentile or below the 5th percentile for the child's age requires further evaluation.

Microcephaly, a small head, may result in severe developmental delay because the brain cannot grow normally. *Macrocephaly,* a large head, may be the result of rapid head growth due to a tumor, or *hydrocephalus,* excessive cerebrospinal fluid within the skull.

Assessment Techniques/ Normal Findings	Special Considerations
3. Assess the child's developmental status. For children under 6 years of age, use a standardized tool such as the Denver II. For older children, assess development by discussing school progress.	Infants and children with suspected developmental delays or learning problems require referral for additional testing. Early identification and intervention promote a better outcome.

Skin, Hair, and Nails

1. Inspect and palpate the skin for general condition. • Note texture, consistency, and temperature. • Gently spread all creases to adequately assess the skin, especially in infants and obese children. • Palpate the skin for dryness, firmness, turgor, and temperature. The skin should be smooth, warm, and even.	Excessive dryness may be due to eczema, overexposure to the sun, or nutritional deficiency. Excessive moisture may indicate perspiration or shock. Poor skin turgor indicates dehydration. Generalized hyperthermia may be seen in children with fever or sunburn. Localized hyperthermia may indicate local infection or burn. Generalized hypothermia may indicate exposure to cold in an infant or shock in an older child.
2. Inspect skin color and pigmentation. • Confirm uniformity of color.	Generalized erythema may be seen in febrile children. Localized erythema may be seen with infection or sunburn. Generalized pallor may indicate shock, circulatory failure, or chronic disease, and requires evaluation.
• Inspect for cyanosis.	Striking cyanosis of the lower extremities may occur in children with coarctation of the aorta. Cyanosis in older infants and children indicates inadequate oxygenation and requires immediate referral.

Assessment Techniques/ Normal Findings	Special Considerations
• Inspect for jaundice.	Jaundice appearing in infants during the first 12 hours of life requires medical treatment. Jaundice may indicate ABO incompatibility, sepsis, hepatitis, or bile duct obstruction.
3. Inspect and palpate the skin for lesions. Note distribution, size, shape, color, and consistency of birthmarks and lesions.	*Mongolian spots* are flat, blue patches usually found on the buttocks or sacral area of infants or young children with dark skin pigmentation. These spots gradually fade.

Capillary hemangiomas appear as flat, pink lesions soon after birth, become raised and red during the first year, then gradually fade.

Impetigo, a common skin infection, may be crusted or bullous; topical or systemic antibiotic treatment is required.

Referral

Suspect child abuse with any of the following diagnostic cues: round or oval bruises on the anterior lower legs, bruises on the face or trunk, bruises that are linear or of an unusual shape or pattern, bite marks, or burns. Obtain medical assistance and follow your state's legal requirements to notify the police or local protective agency. |

Assessment Techniques/ Normal Findings	Special Considerations
4. Inspect the scalp, hair, and nails. Separate hair to inspect the scalp. Note the distribution and texture of the hair on the head and body. The hair should be clean and shiny, generally uniform in color and should cover the head. Infants may normally have areas of baldness on the back and sides of the head.	Oily flakes on the scalp indicate seborrheic dermatitis (cradle cap). Areas of baldness in older infants and children may result from local infection, tinea capitis (ringworm), traction from pulling hair into braids, or hair pulling (self-inflicted or child abuse). Small white spots adhering to the hair shaft indicate pediculosis (head lice). Unlike dandruff, pediculosis nits adhere to the hair. Tufts of hair along the spinal column may indicate a spinal abnormality.

Head, Face, and Neck

1. Inspect and palpate the head. • Observe head shape from all directions.	Premature infants often have long, narrow heads throughout infancy. A flat area of the head may result from an infant lying in one position or from *craniosynostosis*, premature closure of a cranial suture. Referral is indicated.
• Palpate head and suture lines, noting any irregularities such as prominent ridges.	In the first few days of life, some infants have *caput succedaneum*, a large, edematous mass of the scalp, which generally crosses the suture line. *Cephalhematoma* appears similar to caput succedaneum and is normally restricted to one bone. It takes several weeks or longer to resorb.
• Attempt to palpate lymph nodes in occipital region.	Palpable occipital lymph nodes indicate an inflammation or lesion of the scalp.

Assessment Techniques/ Normal Findings	Special Considerations
• In infants, palpate anterior and posterior fontanelles with infant sitting and quiet. Note size. A fontanelle may normally feel full in a crying infant or when the infant is lying down.	Bulging of the anterior fontanelle indicates increased intracranial pressure and requires further evaluation. A depressed fontanelle indicates dehydration. Large fontanelles with separated suture lines may indicate hydrocephalus. A small fontanelle may indicate abnormal head growth.
2. Observe head control and position. Observe head control for strength, steadiness, and position. Head should be held straight and have a full range of motion.	Poor head control after the age of 3 to 4 months may indicate developmental delay, neurologic problems, or muscle weakness. Tremor may indicate a neurologic problem. Head tilt may indicate a hearing or vision deficit, or a muscle contracture.
3. Assess the neck. • To inspect the neck of an infant, place infant first in supine position and then in a prone position. Keep the toddler or older child sitting upright.	Retracting in suprasternal area at upper edge of the sternum may indicate respiratory distress.
• Observe for symmetry, size, shape, and pulsations.	
• Palpate neck to locate trachea and thyroid.	An enlarged or nodular thyroid may indicate disease and requires evaluation.
• Palpate the lymph nodes using both hands, and compare findings. Note the location, size, mobility, consistency, and tenderness of palpable cervical lymph nodes.	Cervical lymph nodes up to 1 cm in diameter that are discrete, movable, and nontender are normal in children up to 12 years of age. Enlarged or tender nodes require further examination of area drained by nodes.

Assessment Techniques/ Normal Findings	Special Considerations

Eyes and Vision

1. Inspect the external eyes.
Observe eyes together, in relation to each other, and separately. Note size and placement. Inspect the lids for movement, shape, and condition.

Wide- or closely set eyes may be a clue to a congenital disorder. Eyes slanting upward are seen in children with Down syndrome.

2. Assess extraocular movements.

• Have the child watch a toy as you move it through the six cardinal directions of gaze.

Inability to move the eye fully through all fields of gaze indicates paralysis of an extraocular muscle. Referral is indicated. Continuous nystagmus, a tremorlike movement, is abnormal.

Strabismus is present if light reflection is not in exactly the same spot on each pupil.

• Shine light into eyes and observe for reflection in exactly the same spot on each pupil.

Strabismus that persists after 6 months of age is abnormal and requires referral. *Amblyopia*, loss of vision in one eye, occurs when strabismus is not corrected during the first few years of life

• Perform the cover-uncover test.

Any movement of the eye when it is uncovered indicates strabismus.

3. Assess the internal eye structures.

• Inspect iris for irregularities. Observe pupils for size, equality, and direct and consensual reaction to light.

Unequal pupils or failure of pupils to react to light may indicate a central nervous system abnormality.

• Hold the ophthalmoscope at +8 to +10, about 12 inches from child, and look for red reflex and any opacities.

Absence of a red reflex is abnormal. Opacities indicate cataracts or other serious conditions.

4. Assess vision.

• Have the infant fixate on and follow a bright toy or face.

An infant who does not follow the toy or face should be referred for a full ophthalmologic examination.

Assessment Techniques/ Normal Findings	Special Considerations
• In children over 3 or 4 years of age, you can use a standard vision test such as Snellen E to evaluate vision.	A difference in visual acuity between eyes requires referral. Visual acuity of 20/40 or less in children 4 years and older requires referral.

Ears and Hearing

1. Inspect the outer ear for structure, placement, and position. Note any difference in structure of ears. Palpate outer ear for consistency. Ears should feel like firm cartilage. Newborns' ears may be flat against the head and feel like thin tissue.

Low-set ears may be associated with congenital anomalies.

Protruding ears may indicate swelling behind the ear or congenital lop-ears.

2. Inspect the opening to the ear canal for wax or discharge. Note color, consistency, and amount. A brownish wax discharge is normal.

A purulent, foul-smelling discharge indicates an inner ear infection with perforation of tympanic membrane or infection of ear canal.

3. Inspect the ear canal and tympanic membrane using an otoscope.
- Straighten ear canal by pulling pinna gently down and out for children younger than 3 years, or up and back in older children. Place hand holding otoscope against child's head before inserting speculum.
- Slowly insert speculum and inspect for foreign bodies, lesions, edema, discharge, and cerumen.

Erythema and edema of the ear canal are seen in otitis externa or swimmer's ear.

Assessment Techniques/ Normal Findings	Special Considerations
• Inspect tympanic membrane. Assess mobility of the tympanic membrane by depressing the pneumatic bulb. Normally, the tympanic membrane "flaps" or moves well.	The tympanic membrane is normally pearly gray, but may be erythematous in a crying or febrile child. A red, bulging tympanic membrane with diffuse light reflex usually signals acute otitis media. Lesions or bubbles on the surface of the tympanic membrane indicate possible trauma or myringitis. A visible fluid level or bubbles behind the tympanic membrane indicate serous otitis media. Decreased or absent movement of the tympanic membrane indicates fluid or pus behind membrane.
4. Assess hearing. Observe if infant or toddler turns in the direction of a bell or clapping hands that are out of the visual field. Test children 4 years and older with an audiometer.	Hearing disorders may cause delays in language, speech, and social development. Parental concern or suspicion about an infant's hearing is sufficient reason for a full hearing evaluation.

Nose and Sinuses

1. Inspect the nose for shape, placement, symmetry, and proportion to other facial features.

• Note any unusual shape, deformity, or asymmetry of the nose and nares, and inflammation or lesions.	
• Note any nasal flaring in infants.	Nasal flaring indicates increased respiratory effort and distress in infants. Because infants breathe through their noses up to 3 months of age, they are predisposed to the compromise of the upper airway.

Assessment Techniques/ Normal Findings	Special Considerations
2. Palpate the nose for irregularities and tenderness. In infants, press each naris closed to evaluate patency.	Smell is not usually evaluated during a routine examination.

Mouth and Throat

1. Observe gums and teeth for color, condition, and hygiene.	Red, swollen, bleeding gums may indicate poor oral hygiene, poor nutrition, or infection. Central and lateral incisor caries usually indicate prolonged bottle feeding. A temporary gray discoloration of the teeth may be seen in children taking liquid iron.
2. Inspect the tonsils and posterior pharynx.	
• Do not use a tongue depressor in cooperative children.	Never use a tongue depressor on a child with suspected epiglottitis.
• Gently depress the tongue and inspect the tonsils and posterior pharynx. Assess the tonsils for size, position, and condition. Normal tonsils may have crypts that look like linear pits. The crypts may trap white debris.	Tonsils are usually not visible in newborns, but they are quite large in preschool and school-aged children. They recede at about age 12. Do not confuse debris with exudate associated with infection and found on tonsillar surface.
• Observe posterior pharyngeal wall for postnasal discharge.	Postnasal discharge from the sinuses may be seen along the posterior pharyngeal wall in children with sinus infections.

Chest and Lungs

1. Inspect the entire chest.	
• Note shape, movement, symmetry and abnormalities. The thoracic cage of a newborn is nearly round.	Protuberance of the sternum indicates *pectus carinatum*. Depression of the sternum indicates *pectus excavatum*. Either may compromise lung expansion, if severe. Chest asymmetry may indicate pneumothorax.

Assessment Techniques/ Normal Findings	Special Considerations
• Note shape, color, and placement of nipples.	Supernumerary nipples occasionally occur along the milk line and are considered normal.
• Note the respiratory depth, rate, and effort.	In infants and children younger than 6 to 7 years, respirations are primarily diaphragmatic or abdominal. Breathing is less regular during infancy than in later childhood. Rapid respirations are seen in infants and children with fever and respiratory or general illness.
	Retracting during inspiration may be supraclavicular, suprasternal, substernal, or intercostal; it is seen in children with increased respiratory effort. A prolonged expiratory phase is seen in obstructive respiratory problems such as asthma.
2. Palpate the chest to evaluate chest expansion, swelling, pain, and respiratory vibration.	
• To evaluate expansion, place palm with fingers spread on each side of chest. Chest expansion is normally symmetric.	Asymmetric expansion indicates unilateral lung abnormality.
• Palpate nipple area for breast tissue, noting the size in relation to age. Normal breast development may begin as early as age 8 or 9 and is most often unilateral. Evaluate breasts in girls by Tanner staging, and perform a full breast examination.	*Gynecomastia*, breast tissue in a pubertal boy, is usually unilateral and temporary, although you need to consider an evaluation for hormonal imbalance.
• Palpate for fremitus by having the child repeat "ninety-nine" while palpating all areas of the chest.	The intensity of fremitus diminishes over areas of lung collapse or pleural effusion. The fremitus intensifies over areas of consolidation.

Assessment Techniques/ Normal Findings	Special Considerations

3. Percuss the chest.

Assess front, sides, and back of chest using indirect percussion over intercostal spaces.

Dullness over lungs is abnormal and may indicate fluid or a mass.

4. Auscultate the lungs.

- Listen first with the unaided ear for any sounds associated with breathing, then with the diaphragm of the stethoscope.
- Compare air exchange, character of breath sounds, and adventitious sounds, and evaluate the character of any coughing. Because infants and children have thin chest walls, their breath sounds are louder and harsher than those of adults. Breath sounds are generally vesicular throughout the lung field.

Rales are heard in children with pneumonia or congestive heart failure. Rhonchi and wheezes that clear with coughing indicate bronchitis. Scattered expiratory wheezing is heard in children with asthma, although absence of wheezing in an asthmatic child may indicate considerably diminished air exchange and distress. Unilateral wheezing, usually on the right side, is indicative of foreign body aspiration.

Cardiovascular System

1. Measure blood pressure.

- Measure blood pressure on all children age 3 or older or on a younger child who is ill, if required.
- Ensure that cuff covers 1/2 to 2/3 of upper arm for accurate reading. The thigh may be used if trauma or an IV line prevents use of the arms.

2. Inspect the chest for visible pulsation.

Note location of any pulsations or any obvious bulges or heaves. The apical impulse is often visible in children with thin chest walls.

A precordial bulge to the left of the sternum signals cardiac enlargement.

Assessment Techniques/ Normal Findings	Special Considerations
3. Palpate the pulses in all extremities for rate, rhythm, and strength.	Absent or diminished femoral pulses suggest coarctation of the aorta.
• Normal heart rates vary with age; the pulse should be strong and equal throughout the body.	
• Gently palpate with fingers to locate apical impulse, or point of maximal impulse (PMI). The PMI in children younger than 4 years is normally felt in the fourth intercostal space just to the left of the midclavicular line. In years 4 to 6, it is found in the fourth intercostal space at the midclavicular line; at 7 years, in the fifth intercostal space at the midclavicular line.	With cardiac enlargement, the PMI moves laterally.
• Palpate chest with ulnar surface of hand, feeling for thrills; note location and timing.	A thrill indicates organic heart disease.
4. Auscultate the heart.	
• Begin with the diaphragm of the stethoscope, then use the bell. Have the child sit upright, then lie supine.	
• Note heart rate and rhythm. At each stop, listen for S_1 and S_2, noting the strength, character, and any split of each sound. Then listen to the systole and diastole for any murmurs, clicks, or snaps. Listen in the diastole for S_3 or S_4.	Sinus arrhythmia is normally heard in children. A venous hum is commonly heard in children and is not pathologically significant.
• Listen to the back for any radiating murmurs.	Murmurs of grade 3 or louder, those associated with a thrill, and those heard during diastole almost always indicate heart disease.

Abdomen

1. Inspect the contour and movement of the abdomen.	A concave appearance in older children may indicate malnutrition.

Assessment Techniques/ Normal Findings	Special Considerations
• With the child supine, note any localized fullness.	A concave appearance in older children may indicate malnutrition.
	Distention may indicate pregnancy in menstruating girls, organomegaly, feces in the bowel, or a tumor.
	Peristaltic waves indicate obstruction or, in young infants, possible pyloric stenosis.
• Inspect the umbilicus, noting any irritation, discharge, or odor. The umbilicus should be clean and dry.	Umbilical discharge in a young infant may indicate a granuloma or infection. Infection is often accompanied by a foul odor.

2. Auscultate the abdomen.
Firmly place diaphragm of stethoscope on abdomen. Listen for peristalsis in all four quadrants. Gurgling bowel sounds are usually heard every 10 to 30 seconds. Before determining that bowel sounds are absent, listen for a full 5 minutes.

High-pitched, tinkling sounds are heard in children with diarrhea or an obstruction.

Absence of bowel sounds indicates paralytic ileus.

3. Percuss all areas of the abdomen systematically.
Use indirect percussion. Use scratch method to further define organ borders. Tympany is heard over most of abdomen. Dullness is heard over liver margin, over a full bladder, or a large mass of feces.

4. Palpate the abdomen twice— first superficially, then deeply.
Palpate any painful area last. Begin at the lower left abdomen, inching up to the left costal margin. Repeat procedure in the midline and then on the right. Note tenderness, lesions, and muscle tone.

When enlarged, the spleen feels like the tip of a nose or thumb below the left costal margin.

All masses other than those identified as feces require further evaluation.

Assessment Techniques/ Normal Findings	Special Considerations

Genitals

1. Inspect the external genitals.

- The child should be supine. Uncover only the area to be examined.
- Note presence and distribution of pubic hair.
- In girls, gently spread the labia majora to inspect the mucous membrane, clitoris, and urethral and vaginal openings. Note any edema, erythema, discharge, or lesions.
- In boys, note penis size and presence of testes in scrotum. Note whether the boy has been circumcised. Inspect the urinary meatus (slitlike in boys) and note any discharge.

2. Palpate the external genitals and inguinal areas.

- In girls, palpate the mons pubis and labia majora for masses.
- In boys, gently attempt to retract the foreskin; do not force. Having the boy sit cross-legged may help. Note any adhesions on circumcised boys.
- Palpate testes for size, consistency, shape, and mobility.

- Palpate inguinal areas of both boys and girls, noting any masses or lymph nodes. Small, moveable lymph nodes in this area are normal for a young child.

Labial adhesions in girls may obscure the vaginal and urethral openings. A foul-smelling vaginal discharge may indicate a foreign body, infection, or poor hygiene.

Any mass of the mons pubis or labia majora is abnormal and requires evaluation.

A testis that cannot easily be brought down into the scrotum of a child over 3 years of age may indicate *cryptorchidism,* or undescended testicle.

The continuous presence of fluid in the scrotum of an infant is likely a hydrocele, which will resorb over time. Intermittent scrotal fluid or a single bulge or mass in the inguinal area indicates an inguinal hernia.

Assessment Techniques/ Normal Findings	Special Considerations

Musculoskeletal System

1. Watch the child move, walk, crawl, and play prior to the examination.
Note any asymmetry, lack of limb use, or favoring of one side. | Limping indicates an abnormality that requires evaluation.

2. Inspect and palpate the upper body.
With the child sitting upright, inspect and palpate clavicles, noting any irregularities. Inspect and palpate surrounding muscles, noting symmetry and strength.
Palpate muscles down both arms, feeling for muscle consistency and irregularities. Inspect palms. | A fracture of the clavicle resulting from birth trauma may be recognized by a hard, fixed mass on the clavicle.

Simian creases may be seen in some normal children, but may indicate Down syndrome.

3. Assess the range of motion of all joints.

4. Inspect and palpate the back.
- Infants may lie prone. School-aged children or adolescents should stand straight.
- Inspect and palpate scapulae, vertebrae, and muscles, noting any asymmetry. Shoulders, scapulae, and hips should be level and the spine straight. | Asymmetry may indicate scoliosis.
- Have the child bend at the waist and note any unilateral fullness. Palpate the spine while the child is bending. | When bending, a unilateral fullness or obvious curvature of the spine indicates scoliosis.

5. Inspect and palpate the hips.
- Note any pain, limitation of movement, or asymmetry. In infants, note symmetry of gluteal skin folds. | Unequal gluteal skin folds may indicate congenital dislocation of the hips.

Assessment Techniques/ Normal Findings	Special Considerations
• Test infants for *Ortolani's sign* of hip dislocation. With the infant supine on a firm surface, place thumbs on the inside of both thighs with fingertips resting over the trochanter muscles. Flex both hips and knees and fully adduct each knee. Normally, nothing is heard or felt.	Unequal or limited adduction may indicate hip dislocation. Ortolani's sign is positive for hip dislocation when a click is heard or felt; it is most reliable in infants less than 4 months old.

6. Inspect and palpate the lower extremities.

• In children who can walk, inspect the leg and foot position while the child is standing.	Genu varum requires evaluation for rickets. Referral is required for genu valgum after 7 to 8 years of age.
• Manipulate ankles and feet to assure that they move easily to a neutral position.	Referral is indicated if feet or ankles cannot be easily straightened.

Neurologic System

1. Assess mental status.

• Assess how the child responds to his or her parents and the examination.	
• Note the child's ability to understand and follow directions. Is the behavior appropriate for the child's age?	
• Note evidence of a short attention span, impulsivity, or hyperactivity.	Impulsive, hyperactive children with short attention spans require evaluation and early intervention to improve their ability to function and to avoid developing a poor self-concept.
• Assess the child's speech.	

Assessment Techniques/ Normal Findings	Special Considerations

2. Assess cranial nerve function.
Cranial nerves II, III, IV, and VI are tested during assessment of the eye. Cranial nerves X and XII are evaluated during examination of the mouth. Table 16.1 provides a summary of techniques for testing cranial nerve function in young children.

TABLE 16.1 Testing Cranial Nerve Function in Young Children

Cranial nerves	Procedures and observations
CN I	Use familiar non-noxious smells such as orange or soap. Not routinely tested.
CN II	Use the Snellen E or Picture Chart to test vision. Test visual fields while immobilizing the head as needed.
CN III, IV, and VI	Move an object through the cardinal points of gaze and have the child follow it with the eyes.
CN V	Observe bilateral jaw strength while the child chews a cookie or cracker.
	Touch the child's forehead and cheeks with cotton and watch the child bat it away.
CN VII	Observe the child's face when smiling, frowning, and crying.
	Ask the child to show the teeth.
	Demonstrate puffed cheeks and ask the child to imitate.
CN VIII	Watch the child turn to sounds such as a bell or whisper.
	Whisper a commonly used word, such as "doggie," behind the child's back and have the child repeat it.
CN IX and X	Elicit the gag reflex.
CN XI and XII	Ask an older child to stick out the tongue and shrug the shoulders or raise the arms.

Assessment Techniques/ Normal Findings	Special Considerations

3. Assess infant reflexes.

- Test for *Babinski sign* by stroking the sole of the foot along the outer edge from heel to toe. The toes should fan and the big toes dorsiflex. This reflex is present during the first 2 years.

  A positive Babinski test in a child older than 2 years suggests a lesion in the extrapyramidal tract.

- Test the *Moro reflex* by abruptly changing the infant's position or jarring the infant. The arms should extend, the fingers fan, the head throw back, and the legs flex weakly. Then the arms should return to center with hands clasped, and the spine and lower extremities should extend. This reflex disappears by 3 to 4 months.

  Asymmetry indicates hemiparesis, clavicle fracture, or injury to the brachial plexus. Persistence beyond 4 months suggests brain damage.

- Test the *palmar grasp reflex* by placing a finger in the infant's palm from the ulnar side. The infant's fingers should curve around it. This reflex disappears by 3 to 4 months.

  Asymmetric grasp indicates paralysis; persistence indicates cerebral disorder.

- Test the *rooting reflex* by stroking one cheek. In response, the head should turn in the same direction. The reflex may disappear at 3 to 4 months or persist for up to 12 months.

  Absence indicates severe neurologic disorder.

- Test the *stepping reflex* by lightly touching the infant's feet to a firm surface. The feet should move up and down as if walking. The reflex disappears by 1 to 2 months.

  Persistence is abnormal.

Assessment Techniques/ Normal Findings	Special Considerations
• Test the *tonic neck reflex* by turning the infant's head to one side. The arm and leg should extend on the side to which the head is turned and flex on the opposite side. The response does not occur each time the head is turned. The reflex appears at about 2 months and disappears at 6 months.	This reflex is abnormal if a response occurs each time the head is turned. Persistence indicates major cerebral damage.
4. Assess deep tendon reflexes. • Assess these reflexes only in school-aged children and adolescents. • Compare the symmetry and strength of reflexes.	Hyperactivity of the reflexes may indicate an upper motor neuron lesion, hypocalcemia, or hyperthyroidism. Decreased or absent reflexes may indicate a lower motor neuron lesion, muscular dystrophy, or paralysis.
5. Assess motor function during the musculoskeletal examination and developmental assessment.	

Common Nursing Diagnoses for Infants, Children, and Adolescents

• **Altered growth and development**—state in which an individual demonstrates deviations in norms from his or her age group
• **Fear**—feeling of dread related to an identifiable source which the child validates
• **High risk for injury**—state in which the child is at risk for injury as a result of environmental conditions interacting with the individual's adaptive and defensive resources
• **Knowledge deficit, child/family**—state in which the child or family does not comprehend, learn, or demonstrate knowledge of health care measures necessary to maintain or improve the health of the child

Common Infant, Child, and Adolescent Health Alterations

Acne vulgaris, asthma, chronic allergic rhinitis, cystic fibrosis, fetal alcohol syndrome, otitis media, physical and sexual abuse of children.

Infant, Child, and Adolescent Physical Assessment Summary

General Appearance and Mental Status

1. Observe physical appearance, body structure, mobility, and behavior.

2. Observe interaction between child and parents.

3. Listen to the child's speech.

Growth and Development

1. Obtain accurate height and weight measurements.

2. Measure the head circumference of children under 2 years of age.

3. Assess the child's developmental status.

Skin, Hair and Nails

1. Inspect and palpate the skin for general condition.

2. Inspect skin color and pigmentation.

3. Inspect and palpate the skin for lesions.

4. Inspect the scalp, hair, and nails.

Head, Face and Neck

1. Inspect and palpate the head.

2. Observe head control and position.

3. Assess the neck.

Eyes and Vision

1. Inspect the external eyes.

2. Assess extraocular movements.

3. Assess the internal eye structures.

4. Assess vision.

Ears and Hearing

1. Inspect the outer ear for structure, placement, and position.
2. Inspect the opening to the ear canal for wax or discharge.
3. Inspect the ear canal and tympanic membrane using an otoscope.
4. Assess hearing.

Nose and Sinuses

1. Inspect the nose for shape, placement, symmetry, and proportion to other facial features.
2. Palpate the nose for irregularities and tenderness.

Mouth and Throat

1. Observe gums and teeth for color, condition, and hygiene.
2. Inspect the tonsils and posterior pharynx.

Chest and Lungs

1. Inspect the entire chest.
2. Palpate the chest to evaluate chest expansion, swelling, pain, and respiratory vibration.
3. Percuss the chest.
4. Auscultate the lungs.

Cardiovascular System

1. Measure blood pressure.
2. Inspect the chest for visible pulsation.
3. Palpate the pulses in all extremities for rate, rhythm, and strength.
4. Auscultate the heart.

Abdomen

1. Inspect the contour and movement of the abdomen.
2. Auscultate the abdomen.
3. Percuss all areas of the abdomen systematically.
4. Palpate the abdomen twice—first superficially, then deeply.

Genitals

1. Inspect the external genitals.
2. Palpate the external genitals and inguinal areas.

Musculoskeletal System

1. Watch the child move, walk, crawl, and play prior to the examination.
2. Inspect and palpate the upper body.
3. Assess the range of motion of all joints.
4. Inspect and palpate the back.
5. Inspect and palpate the hips.
6. Inspect and palpate the lower extremities.

Neurologic System

1. Assess mental status.
2. Assess cranial nerve function.
3. Assess infant reflexes.
4. Assess deep tendon reflexes.
5. Assess motor function during the musculoskeletal examination and developmental assessment.

Chapter 17

Assessing the Childbearing Client

Focused Interview

The first prenatal visit focuses on collection of baseline data about the client and her partner, identification of risk factors, and establishment of a trusting nurse-client relationship. Most of the following questions are appropriate for an initial visit during the first trimester; they expand the information gathered during the complete health history. If the complete health history is not available, be sure to collect this information during the first prenatal visit.

1. What is your age? (Clients under age 15 and over age 35 have increased age-related risks during pregnancy.)
2. Who lives at home with you?

Present Pregnancy

1. What leads you to believe you are pregnant?
2. When was the date of your last menstrual period (LMP)?
3. Describe your usual menstrual cycle.
4. Have you had any cramping, bleeding, or spotting since your LMP?
5. Was this pregnancy planned?
6. Have you experienced any discomfort or unusual occurrences since your LMP?
7. What is your typical food intake in a 24-hour period? What are your food likes and dislikes?
8. What is your regular exercise pattern?
9. What type of health care do you typically receive?
10. Do you have a cat? If so, how do you change its litter? (Toxoplasmosis from infected cat litter may have teratogenic effects on the developing fetus.)
11. How much alcohol, tobacco, and caffeine do you consume each day?

12. Do you use any drugs, such as marijuana, cocaine, or heroin? If so, which ones and how much do you use each day?

Previous Pregnancies and Outcomes

1. Have you been pregnant before? How many times?
2. Have you had any history of spontaneous or induced abortions?
3. Describe any previous pregnancies, including the length of pregnancy, the length of labor, problems during pregnancy, medications taken during pregnancy, prenatal care received, type of birth, your perceptions of the experience, the infant's condition and weight at birth, and whether the infant required additional treatment or special care after birth.
4. Do you attend or plan to attend prenatal education classes?

Gynecologic History

1. Do you experience any discomfort during menstruation? If so, please describe.
2. Have you ever had a vaginal infection or sexually transmitted infection?
3. Have you had any reproductive tract surgery?
4. What birth control method did you use prior to this pregnancy?
5. When was your last Pap smear, and what was the result?

Family Health History

1. Is there a history of genetic or congenital birth defects in your family or your partner's family? If so, please describe.
2. Have any members of your family or your partner's family had any of the following conditions: diabetes mellitus, heart disease, hypertension, kidney problems, multiple gestations, bleeding disorders, or allergies?

Psychosocial Health History

1. Describe your feelings about your pregnancy.
2. Describe how you usually cope with stress.
3. Have you ever had any emotional problems? If so, please describe.
4. How do you think your religious beliefs will affect your pregnancy?
5. How does your partner feel about the pregnancy?
6. Who are your most important support persons?
7. What is your highest educational level?
8. What is your occupation?

Partner's Health History

1. Does your partner have any of the following conditions: congenital or genetic diseases, bleeding disorders, cancer, cardiac disease, diabetes, epilepsy, hepatitis, hypertension, renal disease, or psychiatric problems?
2. How much alcohol and tobacco does your partner consume each day?
3. Does your partner use any drugs, such as marijuana, cocaine, or heroin? If so, which ones and how much?
4. What is your partner's educational level and occupation?
5. What is your partner's blood type and Rh factor?

Physical Assessment

- Gather the following equipment:

centimeter measuring tape	gloves
cervical spatula	pelvimeter
cotton applicators	sphygmomanometer
dipsticks	sterile specimen container
Doppler stethoscope or fetoscope	stethoscope
drape	vaginal speculum
examination light	water-soluble lubricant
glass slides	

- Ask the client to void before beginning the exam to decrease discomfort with the pelvic exam. Instruct the client in providing a clean-catch, midstream urine specimen using a sterile container. Perform a dipstick check for albumin, glucose, ketones, and protein. Send the remaining urine to the lab for urinalysis if this is the first prenatal visit.
- The following blood tests are common at the first prenatal visit: blood type, CBC, Rh status, rubella titer, serologic test for syphilis, sickle-cell anemia screen for clients of African ancestry.
- For clients with a history of IV drug use, sexual intercourse with an IV drug user, or multiple sexual partners, test for hepatitis B and HIV.
- Before assessing the pelvic region, put on gloves. If you notice any skin drainage, blood, or other body fluids, put on gloves before proceeding with the exam.
- Perform a psychosocial assessment at each prenatal visit to assess client's emotional responses to pregnancy.

- It is usual to schedule nine prenatal visits for nulliparous clients and seven for multiparous clients. For the first 28 weeks of pregnancy, assess the client every four weeks. From weeks 28 to 36, schedule client visits every two weeks. From 36 weeks until birth, assess the client weekly.
- During subsequent prenatal assessments, focus on documentation of normal physiologic adaptations, early identification of high-risk symptoms, client teaching and other interventions related to comfort, self-care, and recognition of danger signs of pregnancy. Make evaluations to determine future care.

Assessment Techniques/ Normal Findings	Special Considerations

General Survey

1. Measure client's height and weight.
Take measurements to establish baseline. Client should gain a total of 24 to 28 pounds, an average of 2.7 to 3.1 pounds per month, in the following sequence:

- 2 to 4 pounds during the first trimester
- an additional 11 to 12 pounds during both the second and third trimesters

A gain of 6 pounds or more per month can mean pregnancy-induced hypertension and fluid retention. A gain of less than 2.5 pounds per month can mean insufficient nourishment or insufficient utilization of nutrients.

2. Assess client's general appearance and mental status.

Marked anxiety or apathy may indicate unresolved issues related to acceptance or rejection of the pregnancy.

3. Take client's vital signs.
Assess temperature, pulse, respiration, and blood pressure.

An elevated temperature may be related to a vaginal or urinary tract infection. Slight hyperventilation is caused by the pressure of the uterus on the diaphragm. After 20 weeks, increased blood pressure readings may be associated with pregnancy-induced hypertension (PIH), and decreases may indicate supine hypotensive syndrome.

Assessment Techniques/ Normal Findings	Special Considerations

Skin

1. Observe skin for pigmentary changes associated with pregnancy.
Normal changes include spider nevi, linea nigra, striae gravidarum, and chloasma.

2. Observe skin for vascular markings associated with pregnancy.
Normal markings include angiomas, palmar erythema, and palmar pallor.

Head and Neck

1. Inspect mouth.
Look for hypertrophy of the gingival tissue.

Inflammation of gingival tissue may indicate infection. Paleness of gums may indicate anemia.

2. Palpate thyroid.
Assess for slight hyperplasia after the third month of pregnancy.

Enlargement of the thyroid indicates hyperthyroidism.

The Lungs

1. Inspect, palpate, and percuss chest.
Note diaphragmatic expansion and character of respirations. Observe for symmetric expansion with no retraction or bulging of the intercostal spaces. Later in pregnancy, pressure from the growing uterus produces a change from abdominal to thoracic breathing.

Intercostal space retractions with inspiration, bulging with expiration, or unequal expansion are signs of respiratory distress.

2. Auscultate breath sounds.
Confirm that the lungs are clear in all fields.

Rales, rhonchi, wheezes, rubs, absence of sounds, and unequal breath sounds are signs of respiratory distress.

Assessment Techniques/ Normal Findings	Special Considerations

The Heart

1. Auscultate heart sounds with client supine.
Confirm regular rhythm and rate of from 70 to 90 beats per minute (bpm). Heart rate in pregnancy increases 10 to 15 bpm above baseline. Short, systolic murmurs are due to increased blood volume and displacement of the heart.

Thrills, thrusts, skipped beats, gross irregularity, or gallop rhythm may signal cardiac disease.

Breasts and Axillae

1. Inspect breasts.
Pregnancy-associated changes include enlargement, increased pigmentation of areolae, presence of prominent superficial veins, presence of striae, enlargement of tubercles of Montgomery, and presence of colostrum after the 12th week.

Flat or inverted nipples may interfere with breast feeding.

2. Palpate the breasts for tenderness and nodules.
Breasts become nodular and tingling sensations may be felt during pregnancy.

Abdomen

1. Auscultate bowel sounds.

2. Inspect and palpate abdomen.
Note the appearance of skin, and size and contour of abdomen. Confirm absence of masses.

Palpable masses or nodules may indicate cancer or ectopic pregnancy. A distended bladder and inability to void may indicate urinary retention.

Assessment Techniques/ Normal Findings	Special Considerations

3. Assess fundal height.
Measure distance in centimeters from the top of the symphysis pubis to the top of the fundus.

- At 12 weeks, the fundus is at the symphysis pubis.
- At 20 weeks, the fundus is at the level of the umbilicus.
- After 20 weeks, the fundus approximates the weeks of gestation (eg, a fundal height of 28 cm indicates 28 weeks' gestation).

Increased fundal height is associated with multiple pregnancies, polyhydramnios, and hydatidiform moles. Decreased fundal height is associated with fetal growth retardation, fetal death, and fetal abnormalities. Variations may also indicate an error in calculation of the gestational week.

Extremities

1. Inspect the lower extremities for varicose veins.
Mild varicose veins in later pregnancy are normal.

2. Inspect and palpate extremities for edema.
In the late second and third trimester, edema in the hands and ankles is normal.

Marked edema requires physician referral. Redness, heat, and pain in the legs may indicate thrombophlebitis.

3. Assess patellar reflexes.
Normal response is +2; reflexes should be equal in both extremities.

Referral
Hyperflexia (+3) and clonus are signs of preeclampsia. Refer to a physician.

Pelvic Region

1. Inspect external genitals with client in the lithotomy position.
Wash your hands and put on gloves. Note appearance, pubic hair distribution, and vaginal discharge. The labia should be pink or purplish in color, and there may be a slight increase in white discharge.

Redness or irritation of the external genitals may indicate irritation or infection. Bloody, pink, mucousy, or watery discharge may signal preterm labor. Bloody discharge may also signal placental separation. A yellowish-white discharge may indicate infection.

Assessment Techniques/ Normal Findings	Special Considerations
2. Visualize and inspect cervix. Gently insert prewarmed vaginal speculum until cervix can be visualized. Note position and color. The cervix is a bluish color at 8 to 11 weeks. There should be no lesions or ulcerations. A clear or white odorless discharge is normal.	An infection of the cervix may be present with a thick, purulent discharge of mucus, as with gonorrhea; pinpoint vesicles in a reddened base as with herpes simplex II; profuse whitish bubbly discharge and petechial spots on the vaginal wall as in trichomoniasis; or a thick, white "cheesy" discharge with monilial infection.
3. Obtain a Pap smear if indicated. Remember to swab the endocervix, cervical os, and vaginal pool.	
4. Observe walls of the vagina. Unlock and remove the speculum, observing the walls of vagina as it is withdrawn. Early in pregnancy, the vagina assumes a bluish color. As the pregnancy progresses, the vagina distends and becomes smooth, and there is a localized dryness of the mucosa.	
5. Palpate uterus bimanually.	An extremely retroverted uterus will not be palpable abdominally.
6. Palpate ovaries bimanually.	**Referral** Palpable ovarian cysts require physician referral.
Anus and Rectum	
1. Inspect anus and rectum with client in a lateral position. Lift buttocks and inspect. Mucosa should be pink, intact, and free from lumps, lesions, tears, or discharge.	Hemorrhoids or varicosities of veins around anus and rectum may be present. These are caused by pressure from the gravid uterus and constipation. Masses or nodules may indicate cancer.

Assessment Techniques/ Normal Findings	Special Considerations

Pelvic Adequacy

Physicians or nurses with special preparation may perform an assessment to determine whether pelvic size is adequate for a vaginal birth. See pp. 649-653 in Sims, et al., *Health Assessment in Nursing*.

Assessing the Fetus

1. Ask the client about fetal activity patterns.
The first movement should be felt at 18 weeks in multiparous clients and at 20 weeks in primiparous clients. After 27 to 28 weeks, the client should report more than 10 fetal movements in a 12-hour period.

Referral
Marked decrease in fetal activity, or cessation of movement, may indicate fetal compromise, requiring immediate physician referral.

2. Auscultate fetal heart rate with client in a supine position.
- After 10 to 12 weeks' gestation, the fetal heart rate will be audible with a Doppler and should be assessed at each prenatal visit. After 19 to 20 weeks, an ordinary fetoscope may be used.
- Place Doppler (with conductive gel) on client's abdomen midway between umbilicus and symphysis, in the midline. Move Doppler until you hear the fetal heartbeat.
- Confirm a normal fetal heart rate of 120 to 160 bpm and regular rhythm.

If the fetal heart rate is outside this range, refer to a physician.

3. Assess fetal lie.
Inspect the client's abdomen to determine whether the uterus is longest longitudinally or transversely.

The fetus in a persistent transverse lie or breech will most likely require a cesarean delivery.

Assessment Techniques/ Normal Findings	Special Considerations

4. Assess position and presentation of fetus.
After 32 to 34 weeks, the position, presentation, and attitude of fetus can be assessed through Leopold's maneuvers.

Common Nursing Diagnoses Associated with the Childbearing Client

- **Activity intolerance**—state in which an individual has insufficient physiologic or psychologic energy to endure or complete required or desired daily activities
- **Altered nutrition less than body requirements**—state in which an individual experiences an intake of nutrients insufficient to meet metabolic needs
- **Altered sexuality patterns**—state in which an individual expresses concern regarding her sexuality patterns
- **Anxiety**—vague, uneasy feeling the source of which is often nonspecific or unknown to the individual
- **Constipation**—state in which an individual experiences a change in normal bowel habits, characterized by a decrease in frequency and/or passage of hard, dry stools
- **Fatigue**—overwhelming, sustained sense of exhaustion and decreased capacity for physical and mental work
- **Impaired adjustment**—state in which an individual is unable to modify her lifestyle/behavior in a manner consistent with a change in health status
- **Ineffective individual coping**—state in which an individual is unable to problem-solve or use adaptive behaviors to meet life's demands and roles
- **Knowledge deficit**—state in which the individual/family does not comprehend, learn, or demonstrate knowledge of health care measures necessary to maintain or improve health
- **Sleep pattern disturbance**—state in which the individual experiences a disruption in the amount and/or quality of sleep that interferes with desired lifestyle

Common Childbearing Client Health Alterations

Gestational diabetes mellitus, hyperemesis gravidarum, iron-deficiency anemia, placenta previa, pregnancy-induced hypertension, preterm labor, Rh incompatibility, spontaneous abortion, substance abuse.

Childbearing Client Health Promotion and Education

At the conclusion of the assessment, answer any questions the client may have and provide her with information on potential risk factors during pregnancy, measures to promote a healthy pregnancy, and measures to eliminate or alleviate the discomforts of pregnancy.

Risk Factors During Pregnancy

Advise all antepartal clients to report immediately any of the following signs and symptoms:

- Sudden gush of or leaking fluid from vagina
- Vaginal bleeding
- Temperature above 101° F (38.3° C) and chills
- Abdominal pain or cramps
- Epigastric pain
- Persistent vomiting
- Severe headache
- Dizziness, blurred or double vision, or spots before eyes
- Edema of the hands, face, legs, and feet
- Muscular irritability or convulsions
- Painful urination or decreased urine output
- Absence of or marked decrease in fetal movement

Measures for Promoting a Healthy Pregnancy

You may need to recommend some of the following modifications to the client's usual health practices to help her adjust to the changes of pregnancy:

Breast Care

- Wear a well-fitting support bra with wide nonelastic straps, at least three back hooks, and a cup that covers the entire breast. Keep the nipples dry with nonplastic, lined breast pads.
- Avoid using soap on the nipples.

- If you plan to breastfeed, practice gently rolling and pulling the nipple (unless you have a history of preterm labor).

Rest

- Get at least 8 to 10 hours of sleep each night.
- If possible, plan rest periods during waking hours.
- Teach the client about positioning the body for comfort and safety (eg, resting in the left lateral position), especially in the third trimester.

Nutrition

- Your daily caloric intake should increase by 300 to 500 calories per day.
- Take vitamin, iron, and folic acid supplements as recommended by the physician.
- Monitor weight gain throughout pregnancy.

Exercise

- Monitor your heart rate periodically during exercise. Stop if heart rate increases above 140 bpm.
- Stop exercising if you experience excessive fatigue, dizziness, shortness of breath, abdominal pain, vaginal bleeding, or tingling or numbness in extremities.
- Decrease the intensity of exercise as pregnancy progresses.
- Avoid exercises that require balance.
- Wear loose clothing and supportive shoes and bra.
- Rest in the left lateral position after exercise.

Travel

- The lap portion of a seatbelt should rest below the uterus.
- For every 2 hours of driving, get out of the car and stroll for 10 minutes.
- Avoid flying in the final weeks of pregnancy.

Substance Use

- Stop smoking. Avoid alcohol. Avoid illicit drugs.
- Consult with the physician or nurse before taking any over-the-counter medications.

Occupation

- Plan rest periods during work hours. Elevate the legs whenever possible.
- Do not engage in strenuous physical activity.
- Avoid sitting or standing for long periods of time.
- Avoid environmental toxins and other hazards.

Sexual Activity

- Continue sexual activity throughout pregnancy as desired, except in the presence of vaginal bleeding, ruptured membranes, or signs of preterm labor.
- Recognize that desire may change at different stages of pregnancy because of the effects of changing levels of hormones, fatigue, and physical discomfort.

Childbirth Exercises

- Practice Kegel exercises to increase the strength of the muscles of the pelvic floor.

Measures for Promoting a Comfortable Pregnancy

Vomiting

- Avoid odors that initiate symptoms.
- Eat dry carbohydrates such as crackers or toast before rising in the morning.
- Drink liquids between meals.
- Eat small, frequent meals every 2 to 3 hours.
- Contact a physician if vomiting occurs more than once a day.

Urinary Frequency and Urgency

- Drink at least eight 8-oz. glasses of fluid per day.
- Decrease fluid intake in the evening to prevent nocturia.
- Urinate at least every 2 to 3 hours to prevent stasis.
- Report to the physician immediately any signs of urinary tract infections such as burning on urination, painful urination, or fever.

Heartburn

- Eat small meals every 2 to 3 hours.
- Avoid eating highly seasoned or fried foods.
- Avoid lying down after eating.
- Avoid using sodium bicarbonate. Use an antacid recommended by the physician.

Ankle Edema and Varicose Veins

- Elevate the legs above the hips when sitting.
- Avoid prolonged sitting or standing. Avoid crossing legs.
- Practice dorsiflexion of the foot frequently.
- Wear support hose. Avoid wearing knee-highs or thigh-high stockings.

Hemorrhoids

- Eat foods high in fiber.

- Drink 8 to 10 glasses of fluid per day.
- Avoid straining when having a bowel movement.
- Apply ice packs, warm packs, and ointments as prescribed by the physician.
- Gently reinsert hemorrhoids as necessary.

Constipation

- Consume foods high in fiber.
- Drink 8 to 10 glasses of fluid per day.
- Exercise regularly.
- Establish regular bowel elimination times.
- Use stool softeners as recommended by the physician.

Backache

- Practice the pelvic tilt.
- Avoid lifting heavy objects.
- Use proper body mechanics, especially when lifting, and good posture.
- Avoid wearing high-heeled shoes.

Leg Cramps

- Dorsiflex the affected leg to relieve the cramp.
- Apply a warm towel to relieve the cramp.
- Assess the diet for calcium/phosphorus imbalance.

Faintness or Dizziness

- Avoid lying on the back. Use the left lateral position.
- Change body position slowly, eg, when moving from lying down to sitting or standing.
- Avoid standing for prolonged periods.
- When feeling lightheaded, sit down and place head between legs.

Childbearing Client Physical Assessment Summary

General Survey

1. Measure client's height and weight.
2. Assess client's general appearance and mental status.
3. Take client's vital signs.

Skin

1. Observe skin for pigmentary changes associated with pregnancy.
2. Observe skin for vascular markings associated with pregnancy.

Head and Neck

1. Inspect mouth.

2. Palpate thyroid.

The Lungs

1. Inspect, palpate, and percuss chest.

2. Auscultate breath sounds.

The Heart

1. Auscultate heart sounds with client supine.

Breasts and Axillae

1. Inspect breasts.

2. Palpate the breasts for tenderness and nodules.

Abdomen

1. Auscultate bowel sounds.
2. Inspect and palpate abdomen.

3. Assess fundal height.

Extremities

1. Inspect the lower extremities for varicose veins.
2. Inspect and palpate extremities for edema.

3. Assess patellar reflexes.

Pelvic Region

1. Inspect external genitals with the client in the lithotomy position.
2. Visualize and inspect cervix.
3. Obtain a Pap smear if indicated.

4. Observe walls of the vagina.
5. Palpate uterus bimanually.
6. Palpate ovaries bimanually.

Anus and Rectum

1. Inspect anus and rectum with client in a lateral position .

Assessing the Fetus

1. Ask the client about fetal activity patterns.
2. Auscultate fetal heart rate with client in a supine position.

3. Assess fetal lie.
4. Assess position and presentation of fetus.

Chapter 18

Assessing the Older Adult

Focused Interview

Although elderly people have fewer acute illnesses than younger adults, these illnesses are more serious and more likely to lead to a chronic disorder when they strike. When assessing older adults, keep the following points in mind:

- Call clients by their last name preceded by an appropriate title unless otherwise instructed.
- Begin with clients' concerns and listen carefully to their explanations of their health status and problems, as well as their understanding of their current medical regimen.
- Remember that elderly individuals sometimes tire easily. Plan to complete the assessment in more than one meeting if necessary.
- Allow some time for life review to elicit long-term patterns of functioning and social support. However, refocus the interview if the life review tends to dominate the assessment.
- It is often helpful to get collaborative information from significant others or caretakers, but be sure to include the client in the discussion. Avoid talking about clients in their presence.

Questions for the Client

If there is evidence of possible changes in mental status, direct some questions to caretakers or family members when not in the presence of the client.

1. What would you like help with today?
2. Describe what you do during a typical day.
3. How often do you walk outside? Have you experienced any dizziness when you get up from bed or from a chair?
4. Do you have any problem holding your urine? How many times do you get up at night to urinate?

5. Do you have problems with your bowels? How frequently do you expect to have a bowel movement? What do you do to manage your bowel functioning?

6. Do you know what your medications are and why you are taking them? How long have you been taking each of these medications?

7. Are you having pain or discomfort in any areas of your body? Tell me what this discomfort means for you.

8. Do you have enough energy to do the things you want to do each day?

9. Do you feel you get enough sleep at night? Describe a typical night. What do you do to help yourself go to sleep?

10. Do you have periods when you feel especially sad or lonely? Do you ever feel like you want to end your life?

Questions for Family Members or Caregivers

1. Have you noticed any forgetfulness or changes in the way (the client) normally does things? Has (the client) stopped performing any of his or her normal activities? Have you noticed any unusual behavior?

2. Do you have any concerns about (the client) that you do not want to discuss with him or her?

Physical Assessment

*   Gather the following equipment:

centimeter measuring device	reflex hammer
cotton	safety pins
drape	sphygmomanometer
examination gown	stethoscope
examination light	substances to taste and smell
gloves	tongue blade
ophthalmoscope	tuning fork
otoscope	vision screener
penlight	

*   Warm your stethoscope.
*   Ask whether the client needs to void before the examination.
*   To prevent discomfort due to temperature sensitivity, allow the elderly client to remain clothed, removing only what is necessary to examine a specific area.
*   Whenever possible, conduct the exam in the client's room, with the client on the bed or in a chair.

Assessment Techniques/ Normal Findings	Special Considerations

General Survey and Mental Status

1. Observe the client seated.
Note signs of distress, physical deformity, and so on.

Facial grimacing, pallor, or perspiration could indicate pain or anxiety. A deformity such as "dowager's hump" could indicate the need to probe for pathologic fractures.

2. Observe the client's movements around the examining area.
Observe range of motion, gait, overall mobility, and posture.

Alterations can imply arthritis, neuromuscular disorders, stroke, or degenerative disorders such as Parkinson's disease. However, elderly people tend to slow down and become stooped.

3. Evaluate the client's nutritional status.
Observe for a wasted or apathetic appearance. Measure height and weight and compare findings to height/weight scales for older adults.

Extreme loss of muscle and fat might be due to inadequate nutrition or wasting diseases such as cancer.

4. Observe the client's general hygiene, grooming, and dress.

An unkempt appearance may be a sign of physical inability to care for self, depression or other mental illness, or deteriorating mental functioning. Also, it may be due to abuse and neglect by caregivers.

5. Note the client's interactions with family members or caregivers, and with you.

Excessive passivity or aggression can point to mental dysfunction, a dysfunctional family system, or abuse.

6. Observe client's general attitude, behavior, communication, and ability to follow directions.
Note speech defects, inattention, or failure to comply with spoken or written directions.

These observations can point out hearing or vision disruptions, alterations in mental status, depression, or neurologic disease. Speech problems include aphasia, scanning, or motor speech alterations such as slurring. Inability to follow directions could indicate hearing loss or receptive aphasia from stroke or dementia.

Assessment Techniques/ Normal Findings	Special Considerations

7. Note any breath or body odors.

The odor of urine/ammonia or feces is a sign of incontinence or neglect of personal hygiene; ammonia odor on breath and body may be due to renal failure. Fruity/acetone odor points to ketoacidosis in type I diabetes or starvation.

8. Evaluate mental status.
Use the Mini Mental Status Examination (MMSE) or the Short Portable Mental Status Questionnaire.

These tools can identify subtle changes in memory and judgment that the client could disguise in ordinary conversation by confabulation.

9. Measure vital signs.
- Take the blood pressure in both arms with the client reclining, sitting, and standing. Use a child-sized cuff for very thin, frail persons. Allow a minute or two between each measurement.

Orthostatic hypotension (drop of 20 mm Hg or more) is common.

- Try Osler's maneuver to evaluate for hypertension: Pump cuff above systolic BP to see if the brachial artery is still palpable.

35% to 50% of elderly people have hypertension.

Referral
If the brachial artery is still palpable, pseudohypertension is likely, and the client should be referred to a physician for further evaluation. A diastolic pressure of more than 90 should be watched; referral is required if it persists.

- Take the pulse both apically and radially and compare, checking for pulse deficit. Note if the pulse is irregular, and check for extra or dropped beats.

Arrhythmias are very common and affect the radial pulse. It is helpful to take radial and apical pulses simultaneously to check for pulse deficit, which is common in clients with atrial fibrillation and ventricular ectopic beats. Consider medications as a cause if the pulse is very slow or too fast.

Assessment Techniques/ Normal Findings	Special Considerations
• Take tympanic temperature if possible. Otherwise, take oral temperature. • Observe respirations after listening to apical beat while the stethoscope is still on the client's chest.	Temperature is typically subnormal to low (95 to 97° F) and may not become elevated with infection. Medications may also affect temperature.

Integumentary System

1. Inspect the skin for color. Note any overall redness, cyanosis, jaundice, or pallor. Check for erythema on bony prominences on an immobilized person and in moist areas such as the groin and under the breasts.	Pallor could indicate anemia, malnutrition, or edema. Erythema could indicate an inflammation, irritation, or beginning decubitus ulcer. Differentiate visible veins from cyanosis.
2. Palpate the skin. **Alert!** Put on gloves if open sores or drainage are visible. Note moisture or dryness, scaliness, temperature changes, and texture, especially wrinkling or thinness. Skin loses elasticity with age, so expect some wrinkling and decreased turgor.	*Xerosis* (extreme dryness) is not uncommon, but moisturizers should be used to prevent cracking. Extremely thin, fragile skin, especially in conjunction with under-skin hemorrhages, excessive bruising, and *purpura*, may signal long-term corticosteroid use. In this case, take special care to avoid tearing or other trauma.
3. Measure and describe any skin lesions. • Look for common and non-significant lesions of aging skin: *cherry angiomas, senile lentigos, seborrheic keratoses,* and *skin tags.* Describe and measure these so new lesions or changes can be identified. • Inspect precancerous *actinic keratoses* for cancerous lesions such as melanoma and basal- or squamous-cell carcinomas.	Altered pigmentation, especially in less vascular areas, is not unusual but may represent more easily traumatized tissue. Herpes zoster is more common in older adults; be suspicious of painful, red, vesicular or pustular lesions that have a unilateral dermatome distribution. Ecchymoses, petechiae, or purpura may indicate a bleeding disorder.

Assessment Techniques/ Normal Findings	Special Considerations
• Identify any areas of trauma and potential decubitus or vascular ulcers.	Excessive bruising, burns, or unexplained trauma could be signs of abuse.
4. Inspect the client's hair. Observe amount, distribution and color. Note excessive or total loss of hair; abnormal location of hair, especially gender related; and dry, brittle, or coarse hair.	Expect increased growth of facial hair in women, and more nasal and ear hair in both sexes. Gray or white hair is normal due to loss of melanocytes. Dry, brittle hair may indicate malnutrition or overprocessing. Dull, dry, coarse hair could indicate hypothyroidism.
5. Inspect the nails and nail beds. Note condition, hygiene, nail bed angle, and blanching.	Nails can become thicker or more brittle, but extreme brittleness and tearing could indicate protein deficiency or diabetes. Very thick nails are seen in diabetes and vascular insufficiency. Delayed blanching (longer than 6 seconds) is common with thickened, aging nails and may not be an accurate reflection of circulatory status. Long, dirty nails are a sign of caretaker neglect or inability to care for self. Nail clubbing is related to chronic lung or cardiac diseases.

Head and Neck

1. Observe the face for drooping.	Drooping is usually a sign of stroke or cranial nerve damage.

Assessment Techniques/ Normal Findings	Special Considerations
2. Inspect the eyelids, cornea, and iris. Note the position of the lid on the iris, identifying any tumors or cloudiness of cornea, rings over limbus, irregularities of iris, and inturning or drooping of lids.	Ptosis, especially if unilateral, is a sign of dysfunction of cranial nerves III and IV, possibly due to stroke. Bilateral ptosis may be due to ocular myasthenia gravis. *Pterygium* is not significant, nor is *arcus senilis.* Cloudiness over the iris and pupil could be due to beginning cataracts. Irregularities of the iris may be genetic in origin but more likely is due to previous surgery for glaucoma. *Entropion* and *ectropion* are the result of loss of muscle tone.
3. Check the pupils for size, equality, and reactivity. Ensure room is dimly lighted or client is facing away from sources of outside light. Note both consensual and direct response to light.	Pupils decrease in size with age, so you may have difficulty eliciting pupillary constriction. Lack of consensual response or inequality of size may indicate damage to cranial nerve III. Unusually small pupils (smaller than 2 mm) may be due to ophthalmic miotic medications for glaucoma.
4. Measure visual acuity. Use a hand-held Snellen vision screener. Note if the client holds screener more than 14 inches away in order to read. Loss of accommodation and power, called *presbyopia,* is a normal finding.	Loss of central vision indicates macular degeneration. Blurring or cloudiness could be related to glaucoma, diabetic retinopathy, or cataracts.
5. Check peripheral fields of vision. Note in particular any losses of either left or right fields of vision.	A right or left hemispheric stroke can result in a loss in contralateral visual field. Bilateral loss of peripheral vision may indicate cataracts or glaucoma.

Assessment Techniques/ Normal Findings	Special Considerations
6. Inspect the fundus of the eye with an ophthalmoscope. Note any dark areas in the red reflex, changes in the optic disc, and the appearance of the blood vessels.	Black spots in the red reflex are signs of opacities as may be seen in cataracts. "Cupping" of the disc is a sign of glaucoma, and "fuzzy disc" indicates cerebral edema. Changes of aging include narrower and straighter vessels. Narrowing and tapering of the arterioles are seen in hypersensitive disease, and small red spots or creamy round lesions are punctuate hemorrhages and exudate seen in diabetic retinopathy.
7. Gently palpate the eyeball. Ask the client to close eyes. Gently palpate. Note tension or firmness.	Very soft or boggy eyeballs indicate dehydration, whereas rock-hard orbits could mean glaucoma.
8. Evaluate the client's hearing. Use the whisper, Rinne, and Weber tests; use a 512 or 1024 tuning fork.	Hearing loss with aging begins with diminished perception of high-frequency sounds. In sensorineural hearing loss, the Rinne test is normal, but the Weber test shows the sound lateralizing to the good ear or equal in both if hearing is diminished bilaterally.
9. Inspect the outer ear, ear canal, and tympanic membrane. Use an otoscope to inspect the ear canal and ear drum. Note any excessive earwax or changes in the tympanic membrane.	Excessive wax may cause a conductive hearing loss. Scarring and sclerosis of tympanic membrane from repeated inflammation or infection give a darkened appearance or dark lines.
10. Evaluate the client's sense of smell. Use easily identified substances such as cloves or lemon.	Smell and taste diminish with age, but perceiving unusual odors may be a sign of temporal lobe epilepsy. An inability to distinguish pungent, common odors could be related to neurologic dysfunction such as stroke.

Assessment Techniques/ Normal Findings	Special Considerations

11. Inspect the oral mucous membranes, gums, throat, and tongue.

- Note color, exudate, swelling, and lesions.

White patches could be precancerous leukoplakia. If the client is wearing dentures, redness and leukoplakia are signs that they fit poorly.

A dark red, swollen tongue with white or yellow adherent patches is a sign of fungal infection, which older people on antibiotics commonly experience.

- Have the client say "ah" as you depress the tongue with a tongue blade. Check for symmetric elevation of the soft palate.

Unequal elevation or loss of elevation of the soft palate occurs with impairment of cranial nerves IX and X, seen with stroke. In this case, the client is at risk for choking and aspiration.

12. Palpate and auscultate the carotid arteries.
Proceed gently, palpating one artery at a time. Auscultate with the bell of the stethoscope. Note any bruits.

Bruits are signs of carotid stenosis and impending stroke. If you hear bruits, check the aortic and pulmonic valve areas of the chest for murmurs, which may be radiating into the neck.

13. Inspect and palpate the neck vein.
Assess veins first with client lying flat and then with client elevated above 45 degrees. Note any firmness and distention.

Veins are normally soft and compressible. If they are flat when the client is supine, suspect dehydration. If neck veins are visible, firm to the touch, or tortuous when the client is elevated 45 degrees, suspect venous pressure and right heart failure.

Assessment Techniques/ Normal Findings	Special Considerations
14. Evaluate the range of motion of the neck.	Limited range of motion in the neck is often related to cervical arthritis, degenerative disc disease, or muscle spasm. If *kyphosis* is present, hyperextension of the neck is difficult.

Heart and Lungs

1. Take the apical pulse. Note rate, rhythm, and irregularities. Arrhythmias are quite common in healthy elders.	Abnormally slow rates could indicate heart block or sinus arrest, especially if accompanied by syncope. Fast or grossly irregular rhythms point to potentially serious tachyarrhythmias, especially if accompanied by chest pain or dizziness. After periods of immobilization, increased heart rate can indicate decompensation.
2. Auscultate the precordium. • Check for murmurs, clicks, and S_3 or S_4 gallops. • Using the bell of the stethoscope, listen for low-pitched murmurs during S_3 and S_4. Holosystolic, grade III without radiation, and S_3 murmurs are common in older people because of decreased cardiac muscle tone. • Using the diaphragm, listen for high-pitched murmurs, clicks, and snaps. If you hear a murmur, inch the stethoscope away from the site in several directions to check for radiation. Describe murmurs using specified criteria (see Chapter 8).	Loud murmurs of grade IV or greater and with thrills and/or radiation suggest a failing heart, or valvular stenosis or incompetency. Murmurs that radiate from the base near the sternal border, right or left, up into the neck, are usually related to aortic or pulmonic valve disease. Clicks and snaps are opening sounds and point to aortic or mitral calcifications. A fixed splitting of the second heart sound (throughout the respiratory cycle) is noted in pulmonary hypertension or chronic obstructive pulmonary disease.

Assessment Techniques/ Normal Findings	Special Considerations
3. Inspect the shape of the thorax. Look for increased anteroposterior diameter and spinal curvature abnormalities that may affect respiration.	Severe barrel chest is a sign of chronic obstructive pulmonary disease. Also, kyphosis and scoliosis may decrease lung expansion.
4. Inspect and palpate the chest walls and ribs. • Assess pain or tenderness to touch, crepitus, or bruising.	Pain upon palpation of the ribs is a sign of pathologic rib fractures, which can occur in clients with osteoporosis without any major trauma. Also look for bruising in conjunction with rib pain, which could be due to falls or physical abuse.
• Palpate for tactile fremitus.	Increased fremitus, especially in the periphery, indicates fluid accumulation or tissue consolidation.
5. Percuss the lung fields. Check for hyperresonance or dullness.	Anticipate hyperresonance in the older adult with chronic obstructive pulmonary disease. Dullness indicates fluid accumulation from pulmonary edema or retained secretions. Dullness could also indicate tissue consolidation from a tumor or mass.
6. Auscultate the lung fields. Note the characteristics of sounds, decreased aeration or expansion, adventitious sounds such as rales or wheezes, and altered vocal resonance.	Rales that extend upward and do not clear with a cough suggest pulmonary edema. Coarse, loud rales may be signs of pulmonary fibrosis, seen in people with long-standing lung disease. If the person has increased trapped air from emphysema, breath sounds and vocal resonance will be diminished. Difficulty hearing any breath sounds, harsh rhonchi, or bronchiovesicular breath sounds in the periphery indicate advanced chronic lung disease.

Assessment Techniques/ Normal Findings	Special Considerations

Breast

1. Inspect and palpate the female and male breasts.
Note changes in symmetry, lumps or thickening of tissue, lesions or sores, inflammation, changes in nipples, or drainage from open lesions or from nipples.

Hormonal changes can increase breast tissue in males and put them at risk for breast cancer. Females on postmenopausal hormone therapy are also at increased risk for breast cancer, especially if female relatives have had it. Early identification of tumors is vital.

Abdomen

1. Inspect the abdomen.
Observe for shape, symmetry, pulsations, and visible tortuous veins, especially near the umbilicus.

A flaccid or "potbelly" abdomen is common because of loss of collagen and muscle, and deposition of fat.

Asymmetry may indicate tumors, hernia, constipation, or a bowel obstruction.

Lateral pulsations or soft, pulsatile masses in the aorta indicate an aortic aneurysm.

Visible tortuous veins on the abdominal wall near the umbilicus, in conjunction with a firm and distended abdomen, indicate portal hypertension with ascites.

2. Auscultate the abdomen.
• Note the number and quality of bowel sounds.

Bowel sounds may be hypoactive. Borborygmi may be due to bleeding or inflammatory bowel disease. High-pitched hyperactive bowel sounds accompanied by colicky pain and distention are signs of small bowel obstruction, which occurs most often in elderly men.

• Check for vascular bruits over the aorta, in flank areas for renal arteries, and over both groins for femoral and iliac arteries.

Bruits heard over any of the arteries are signs of stenosis or aneurysms.

Assessment Techniques/ Normal Findings	Special Considerations
3. Percuss the abdomen. • Note tympany and dullness over most of the abdomen.	Areas of dullness in the lower left quadrant and sigmoid area are probably related to stool, but tumors must be ruled out.
• Check for shifting dullness.	Shifting dullness, especially when accompanied by firm dullness, suggests ascites.
4. Palpate the abdomen. • Note tenderness, firmness, rigidity, and masses.	Firmness is associated with fluid or excessive gas, but rigidity is a sign of peritoneal inflammation.
	Distention just above the symphysis pubis may be caused by bladder distention due to prostatic hypertrophy or incomplete emptying.
• Palpate the costal margin at the right midclavicular line and the midsternal line for liver enlargement.	If the liver is palpable below costal margins, the liver is probably enlarged. Enlargement may reflect passive congestion due to congestive heart failure or liver disease, especially if liver feels nodular.

Genitourinary System

Female

1. Check the underclothing for staining. If present, note color and odor.	Staining indicates incontinence or vaginal discharge.
2. Inspect the external genitals. Note changes in tissue, redness, swelling, or odor. Atrophy of the labia is usual.	Redness, swelling, or odor can indicate incontinence, yeast infections, inadequate self-care, or caregiver neglect. A fecal odor could signal a urinary tract infection.

Assessment Techniques/ Normal Findings	Special Considerations
3. Perform a pelvic examination. Assist the client into a left lateral decubitus position. Perform the examination in the client's bed if possible.	Bulging of tissue or muscle into the vagina or rectum indicate cystocele, rectocele, or uterine prolapse. Vaginal atrophy and dryness may make examination painful. Malodorous vaginal discharge could be a sign of cancer or infection.
4. Examine the rectum. Note sphincter control. Check for hemorrhoids. Take a stool sample and check for occult blood.	Sphincter control decreases with age, resulting in incontinence. Rectal cancer is more common in older people; occult blood in the stool is a fairly early sign.

Male

1. Check the underclothing for staining. Note color and odor of any stains.	Staining indicates incontinence. Small amounts of dried blood could indicate intermittently bleeding hemorrhoids.
2. Examine the external genitals. Observe for swelling, redness, or odor.	Testicular atrophy is normal, but swelling could be a sign of infection or prostatic hypertrophy. Swelling, redness, and odor can be a sign of infection, incontinence, poor self-care, or caregiver neglect.
3. Perform a rectal exam. Note sphincter control. Check for prostate enlargement and any rectal abnormalities such as hemorrhoids. Take a stool sample and check for occult blood.	Prostatic hypertrophy can be benign or malignant; encourage the client to get a PSA (prostate-specific antigen) test. Elevated levels usually indicate carcinoma of the prostate. The occult blood test can detect colon cancer, which increases in incidence in men over 40. Hemorrhoids can cause bright red bleeding as well as a red stain in the stool. A mass in the rectum could be rectal cancer.

Assessment Techniques/ Normal Findings	Special Considerations

Musculoskeletal System

1. Inspect and palpate the spinal column with the client seated. Note abnormal curvatures, deformities, pain, or tenderness with palpation of vertebrae, and bruising or other signs of trauma.

Shortening of the spine due to flattening of the discs is very common. Loss of bone matrix and decreased muscle mass and tone can result in increased curvatures such as kyphosis, lordosis, or scoliosis. Arthritis and degenerative disc disease can cause spinal deformities.

Pain upon palpation of vertebrae and generalized back pain indicate pathologic fractures due to osteoporosis. Bruising or unusual lesions on the back could indicate falls or physical abuse.

2. Inspect and palpate all joints. Assess for pain, heat, redness, swelling, deformity, and range of motion.

Heat, redness, swelling, and pain on movement of joints indicates bursitis or gouty or septic arthritis. Osteoarthritis causes swelling and joint deformity with early morning stiffness and pain. Hands and weight-bearing joints, such as hips and knees, are most often affected.

3. Inspect and palpate the feet. Note color, skin integrity, any deformities, and signs of inflammation, infection, or ulcerations. Palpate pedal pulses.

The inability to palpate pulses, especially if the feet are red or dusky in color, indicates arterial insufficiency.

Pitting edema of the feet and legs due to venous incompetency or right-sided heart failure may be present.

Assessment Techniques/ Normal Findings	Special Considerations

Neurologic System

1. Evaluate balance and coordination.
- Assess the client's ability to walk heel-to-toe forward and backward.
- Have the client perform the Romberg test with eyes closed. Stand next to the client to catch if necessary. If the client begins to lose balance, have the client open eyes.

The heel-to-toe walk is often impaired and does not indicate any specific disease, but it can place the person at risk for falls. Falling forward and a propulsive gait indicate Parkinson's disease. If the client has good balance with eyes open, the defect is probably proprioceptive rather than of basal ganglion or cerebellar origin.

2. Inspect for tremors of the head, face, and extremities.
Note the type of tremor and whether it is present at rest or primarily occurs with movement.

Senile (gross) tremors of the head, jaw, and tongue are not treatable. Resting tremors diminish with willed movement. A pill-rolling tremor of the hand is seen in Parkinson's disease. People taking bronchodilator drugs have a fine tremor that increases with activity.

3. Evaluate motor strength.
- Assess the client's arm drift. Have the client stand with feet comfortably apart, and arms held straight out at shoulder level. Check arm drift first with the client's eyes closed, then open.
- Assess the client's grip and extremity strength against resistance. Inspect the muscles for size, comparing one side with the other. Palpate the muscles for tone.

Subtle hemiparesis is indicated by a slow downward drift and pronation of the hand on the affected side when the eyes are closed; if the client is able to correct the drift when the eyes are opened, suspect proprioceptive dysfunction.

Unilateral diminished grip and loss of strength against resistance can indicate a stroke. Loss of innervation to specific muscle groups or paralysis from stroke or other neurologic diseases results in atrophy and loss of or increased tone.

Assessment Techniques/ Normal Findings	Special Considerations
4. Evaluate sensation. Ask the client to sit and close eyes. Check various sites for sensitivity to touch and vibration. Assess stereognosis. Evaluate proprioception by having the client identify the position to which you move a toe or finger.	Suspect a neurologic disease such as cerebrovascular accident if sensation is absent in any area, especially unilaterally. Diminished or absent sensation symmetrically in the lower extremities is a sign of diabetic peripheral neuropathy.
5. Evaluate the reflexes with a reflex hammer. Note diminished or increased reflexes.	Reflexes normally diminish with aging. If they are absent, suspect upper motor neuron disease; if they are hyperactive, especially with clonus, suspect lower motor neuron disease.

Common Nursing Diagnoses for the Older Adult

- **Activity intolerance**—state in which an individual has insufficient physiologic or psychologic energy to endure or complete required or desired daily activities
- **Altered health maintenance**—inability to identify, manage, or seek out help to maintain health
- **Altered nutrition**—state in which an individual experiences an intake of nutrients insufficient to meet metabolic needs
- **Body image disturbance**—disruption in the way one perceives one's body image
- **Caregiver role strain**—a caregiver's felt difficulty in performing the family caregiver role
- **Chronic pain**—state in which the individual experiences chronic pain that continues for more than 6 months
- **Diversional activity deficit**—state in which an individual experiences a decreased stimulation from or interest or engagement in recreational or leisure activities
- **Fatigue**—overwhelming, sustained sense of exhaustion and decreased capacity for physical and mental work
- **High risk for injury**—state in which the individual is at risk of injury as a result of environmental conditions interacting with the individual's adaptive and defensive resources
- **Home maintenance management**—inability to independently maintain a safe, growth-producing immediate environment

- **Impaired social interaction**—state in which an individual partici-
  pates in an insufficient, excessive, or ineffective quantity of social
  exchange
- **Ineffective family coping**—usually supportive primary person is
  providing insufficient, ineffective, or compromised support, comfort,
  assistance or encouragement that may be needed by the client to
  manage or master adaptive tasks related to his or her health chal-
  lenge
- **Low self-esteem**—negative self-evaluation/feelings about self that
  develop in response to a loss or change in an individual who previously had a positive self-evaluation
- **Perceived constipation**—state in which an individual makes a self-
  diagnosis of constipation and ensures a daily bowel movement
  through use of laxatives, enemas, and/or suppositories
- **Self-care deficit**—state in which an individual experiences an
  impaired ability to perform or complete activities of daily living
- **Stress incontinence**—state in which an individual experiences a loss
  of urine of less than 50 ml occurring with increased abdominal pressure

Common Older Adult Health Alterations

Arthritis, cancer, congestive heart failure, constipation, diabetes, depression and suicide, drug and alcohol abuse, fractures.

Older Adult Client Education

Following are some general suggestions to promote better health in any
older client. Be sure to include any physician-prescribed regimen in
your plan.

Exercise

- Walking, swimming (for people with arthritis or other joint problems), bicycling, low-impact aerobics, and tai chi chuan are all good
  choices of exercise for older adults. Be sure to warm up before any
  exercise, with stretches and low-intensity forms of the exercise.
- Learn what your target heart rate is and how to monitor your heart
  rate during activity.

Hygiene and Skin Care

- Daily bathing may not be necessary, especially if you have excessively dry skin and itching. If you use oil, be sure to rinse all the oil out
  of the tub to prevent slips and falls.

- Inspect your skin and feet for any new lesions, accidental injury, or changes in existing skin lesion, such as changes in the color of moles. See a doctor if you notice anything suspicious.

Medications

- Keep a list of current medications, dosages, and the physician who ordered them. Take the list with you to any doctor appointments, hospital admissions, or outpatient testing. Review the need for the medications or the need for lab testing with the primary physician at least every six months or whenever your health status changes. Give a copy of the list to a family member or friend. Update it as needed.
- Use a medication box and fill it weekly. This is a good way to separate medications taken at different times of the day and to keep track of medications and check if they were all taken.
- Check medications for expiration dates with each refill or monthly for those you take infrequently.
- Know the adverse reactions and side effects of medications; consult with a nurse or physician if you are concerned.
- Wear a medic-alert bracelet or medallion for any diseases or medications that could affect care to be given during an emergency.

Safety

- Keep a list of emergency numbers by the phone or program a memory phone to dial important numbers for you.
- Be sure your smoke alarms are working and keep a fire extinguisher handy.
- If you live alone, leave a house key with a trusted relative, friend, or neighbor.
- Improve the safety of your home by removing obstacles you can trip over, replacing throw rugs with wall-to-wall carpeting or tacked-down rugs, installing handrails in the bathroom, putting nonslip decals in the bottom of the tub or shower, and placing frequently used objects in the same location.

Sexuality

- There is no reason not to enjoy sexual activity. If overt sexual function is not possible, cuddling and touching can still bring pleasure.
- Sexual response is slowed with aging, so be patient with your partner.
- Some medications and diseases impair sexual functioning. Consult with a physician regarding a possible change of medication.

Elimination

- For stress incontinence or dribbling, women can benefit from Kegel exercises.

- If you are taking diuretics, try taking them in the morning. Try to take the last dose before dinner to reduce the number of times you need to get up during the night.
- For constipation, increase activity, fiber in the diet, and water intake. Consult a physician if constipation is not resolved, especially if nausea, vomiting, or abdominal pain accompanies the constipation.
- Take bulk medications to improve elimination, but avoid cathartics.
- Avoid large-volume water enemas because they can complicate the problem of constipation. If you have persistent constipation, use a small-volume "salt" enema, but only occasionally.

Older Adult Physical Assessment Summary

General Survey and Mental Status

1. Observe the client.
2. Observe the client's movements around the examining area.
3. Evaluate the client's nutritional status.
4. Observe the client's general hygiene, grooming, and dress.
5. Note the client's interactions with family members or caregivers and with you.
6. Observe the client's general attitude, behavior, communication, and ability to follow directions.
7. Note any breath or body odors.
8. Evaluate mental status.
9. Measure vital signs.

Integumentary System

1. Inspect the skin for color.
2. Palpate the skin.
3. Measure and describe any skin lesions.
4. Inspect the client's hair.
5. Inspect the nails and nail beds.

Head and Neck

1. Observe the face for drooping.
2. Inspect the eyelids, cornea, and iris.
3. Check the pupils for size, equality, and reactivity.
4. Measure visual acuity.
5. Check peripheral fields of vision.
6. Inspect the fundus of the eye with an ophthalmoscope.
7. Gently palpate the eyeball.
8. Evaluate the client's hearing.
9. Inspect the outer ear, ear canal, and tympanic membrane.
10. Evaluate the client's sense of smell.

11. Inspect the oral mucous membranes, gums, throat, and tongue.
12. Palpate and auscultate the carotid arteries.
13. Inspect and palpate the neck vein.
14. Evaluate the range of motion of the neck.

Heart and Lungs

1. Take the apical pulse.
2. Auscultate the precordium.
3. Inspect the shape of the thorax.
4. Inspect and palpate the chest walls and ribs.
5. Percuss the lung fields.
6. Auscultate the lung fields.

Breasts

1. Inspect and palpate the female and male breasts.

Abdomen

1. Inspect the abdomen.
2. Auscultate the abdomen.
3. Percuss the abdomen.
4. Palpate the abdomen.

Genitourinary System

Female

1. Check the underclothing for staining.
2. Inspect the external genitals.
3. Perform a pelvic examination.
4. Examine the rectum.

Male

1. Check the underclothing for staining.
2. Examine the external genitals.
3. Perform a rectal exam.

Musculoskeletal System

1. Inspect and palpate the spinal column with the client seated.
2. Inspect and palpate all joints.
3. Inspect and palpate the feet.

Neurologic System

1. Evaluate balance and coordination.
2. Inspect for tremors of the head, face, and extremities.
3. Evaluate motor strength.
4. Evaluate sensation.
5. Evaluate the reflexes with a reflex hammer.

llustration and Photo Credits

CHAPTER 4   4.1: Richard Tauber.

CHAPTER 5   5.1: Romaine LoPrete. 5.2, 5.3, 5.4, 5.5: Kristin N. Mount. Table 5.1, Table 5.2: Kristin N. Mount.

CHAPTER 6   6.1, 6.3: Romaine LoPrete. 6.2: Don Wong/Photo Researchers/Nea Hanscomb. 6.4: Richard Tauber/Nea Hanscomb.

CHAPTER 7   7.1, 7.2, 7.3, 7.4, 7.5: Richard Tauber/Nea Hanscomb. 7.3: Romaine LoPrete.

CHAPTER 8   8.1: Dr. Michael Hawke. 8.2: Richard Tauber. 8.3: Romaine LoPrete. 8.4: Richard Tauber/Nea Hanscomb.

CHAPTER 9   9.1: Richard Tauber/Nea Hanscomb. 9.2: Kristin N. Mount. 9.3: Richard Tauber.

CHAPTER 10   10.1: Romaine LoPrete. 10.2, 10.3, 10.4: Richard Tauber/Nea Hanscomb. 10.5, 10.6: Richard Tauber.

CHAPTER 11   11.1: Richard Tauber/Nea Hanscomb.

CHAPTER 12   12.1, 12.2: Richard Tauber. 12.3, 12.4, 12.5, 12.6, 12.7, 12.9, 12.10: Kristin N. Mount. Table 12.1: Romaine LoPrete.

CHAPTER 13   13.1, 13.2, 13.3, 13.4: Richard Tauber. Table 13.1: Romaine LoPrete.

CHAPTER 14   14.1, 14.2, 14.3, 14.4: Richard Tauber/Nea Hanscomb.

CHAPTER 15   15.1, 15.2, 15.3, 15.4: Richard Tauber. 15.5: Romaine LoPrete.

Index

Abdomen
  cardiovascular system assessment and, *98*
  urinary system assessment and, *135*
Abdomen assessment, *120-132*
  in childbearing client, *242-243*
  common alterations found, *131*
  focused interview in, *120*
  in infants, children, and adolescents, *226-227*
  nursing diagnoses in, *130*
  in older adult, *263-264*
  physical assessment in, *121-130, 132*
Abdominal quadrants, organs of, *123*
Abdominal reflexes, assessment techniques/normal findings, *208*
Abdominal sounds, *124, 125*
Abducens nerve, assessment techniques/normal findings, *199-200*
Accessory nerve, assessment techniques/normal findings, *201*
Accommodation, assessment techniques/normal findings, *62*
Achilles tendon reflex, assessment techniques/normal findings, *207-208*
Actinic keratoses, *256*
Activities of daily living (ADLs), *17-19*
Adolescents
  assessment, *212-236*
    physical, *213-233*
  common health alterations found, *234*
  interviewing, *212*
  nursing diagnoses for, *233*
Adventitious sounds, *86, 87*
Affect, physical assessment and, *35*
Air trapping, pattern and causes, *80*
Alcohol use, self-care assessment and, *20*
Amblyopia, *220*
Anemia, *51, 241, 256*
Aneurysm, *97, 99*
  aortic, *98, 122, 129, 137, 263*
  dissecting ascending, *101*
  left ventricular, *99*
Ankles
  assessment techniques/normal findings, *189-191*
  edema, childbearing client and, *249*
Anosmia, *199*
Anus, assessing in childbearing client, *244*
Anxiety, physical assessment and, *35*
Aorta, palpation, *129*
Aortic aneurysm, *98, 122, 129, 137, 263*
Aortic regurgitation, *95, 100*
Aortic stenosis, *99*
Apical pulse, *103*
  assessing in older adult, *261*
Appearance
  assessing in childbearing client, *240*
  assessing in infants, children, and adolescents, *214-215*

physical assessment and, *34-36*
urinary system assessment and, *134-135*
Arcus senilis, *258*
Areolae, palpation, *115*
Arms, peripheral vascular/lymphatic system assessment and, *169-170*
Arrhythmias, *226, 255*
Arteriosclerosis, *51*
Arthritis, *70, 71, 180, 266*
  gouty, *189*
  rheumatoid, *182, 189, 190*
Ascites, *126, 130*
Asystole, *101*
Ataxic breathing, pattern and causes, *80*
Atelectasis, *127*
Atherosclerosis, *93, 96, 103*
Atrial septal defect, *99*
Atrophy, *48*
Auditory canal, assessment techniques/normal findings, *65-66*
Auricle, assessment techniques/normal findings, *65*
Auscultation, *29-30*
Axillae assessment, *109-119*
  in childbearing client, *242*
  common alterations found, *116*
  focused interview in, *109-110*
  nursing diagnoses in, *116-117*
  physical assessment in, *110-116, 119*
Axillae client education, *117-119*
Axillary temperature, *38*

Babinski sign, *232*
Backache, childbearing client and, *250*
Balance, assessment techniques/normal findings, *202*
Baldness, *50, 218*
Bartholin's glands, assessment techniques/normal findings, *156*
Bathing skills, *17-18*
Behavior, physical assessment and, *35*
Belief systems
  organizing data, *16*
  psychosocial health assessment and, *15*
  psychosocial wellness and, *10*
Biceps reflex, assessment techniques/normal findings, *205-206*
Biographic data, *6*
Biot's respirations, pattern and causes, *80*
Birth history, *213*
Bladder infection, preventing, *139*
Blood pressure
  assessing in infants, children, and adolescents, *225*
  assessment techniques/normal findings, *168*
  measuring, *39*
Blumberg sign, *130*
Body build, physical assessment and, *35*